NOT BROKEN
ALLI BALDOCCHI

NOT BROKEN

How My Son with Autism Taught Me to Live

ALLI BALDOCCHI

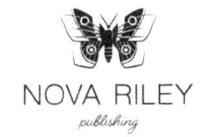

NOVA RILEY
publishing

MANHATTAN BEACH, CA

Copyright © 2020 Alli Baldocchi

All rights reserved. No part of this book may be reproduced or transmitted in any form or by any means, electronic or mechanical, including photocopying, recording, or by an information storage and retrieval system—except by a reviewer who may quote brief passages in a review to be printed in a magazine, newspaper or on the Web—without permission in writing from the publisher.

Nova Riley Publications
Manhattan Beach, CA 90266
www.AlliBaldocchi.com
www.NovaRileyPublishing.com
www.Velcro-Shoes.com

ISBN 978-1-7342114-0-5 print book
ISBN 978-1-7342114-1-2 e-book

Cover photo: Liz Lonky, Life Iz Photography
Cover & Interior Design: Shannon Bodie, www.BookwiseDesign.com

This book is available at quantity discounts for bulk purchase.
Contact the publisher.

**A portion of the proceeds of this book
will be donated to Autism Awareness.**

Publisher's Cataloging-In-Publication Data
(Prepared by The Donohue Group, Inc.)

Names: Baldocchi, Alli, author.
Title: Not broken : how my son with autism taught me to live / Alli Baldocchi.
Description: Manhattan Beach, CA : Nova Riley Publishing, [2020] | Includes
    bibliographical references.
Identifiers: ISBN 9781734211405 (print) | ISBN 9781734211412 (ebook)
Subjects: LCSH: Baldocchi, Alli--Family. | Parents of autistic children--Psychology.
    | Autistic children--Care--Psychological aspects. | Self-actualization
    (Psychology) | Identity (Psychology)
Classification: LCC HQ773.8 .B35 2020 (print) | LCC HQ773.8 (ebook) | DDC
    649/.15--dc23

Printed in the United States of America.

DEDICATION

This book is dedicated to my husband, Tome.

Thank you for your unconditional love and support. Thank you for never questioning or second-guessing the decisions I make and trusting me wholeheartedly. Thank you for standing by me, and always cheering me on. Thank you for giving me the strength and courage to follow my heart and face my truths. Thank you for making me see what has always been. Thank you for being on this journey with me. Watching our boys explore the world and discover who they are and who they want to be, is my happiness. Sharing it with you is my everything.

CONTENTS

	FOREWORD	ix
	ACKNOWLEDGMENTS	xiii
	MY THREE SONS	xix
	INTRODUCTION	1
ONE	MOM IDENTITY	9
TWO	DAD CAN FIX IT	21
THREE	IT TAKES A VILLAGE	27
FOUR	A GIFT OF EMPOWERMENT	39
FIVE	I AM CADEN	51
SIX	WHAT'S THE DEAL WITH THE GUT?	55
SEVEN	FINDING THE LIGHT	69
EIGHT	QUEEN OF THE CASTLE	87
NINE	LITTLE BOY WONDER	95
TEN	MY BROTHER CADEN	107
ELEVEN	CADEN FOR PRESIDENT	111
TWELVE	I'M THE BIG BROTHER	123
THIRTEEN	TURNING POINT	127
FOURTEEN	HOPE & LOVE	135
	GLOSSARY	137
	RESOURCES	145
	ABOUT THE AUTHOR	159

FOREWORD

With the prevalence of Autism Spectrum Disorder (ASD; Autism) rising to one in fifty-nine according to a recent study conducted by the Centers for Disease Control, you are hard pressed to find someone who does not have a story. Colloquial terms such as "ASD," "Autism," or "on the spectrum" have evolved and are casually thrown around in everyday encounters. You often hear, "I have a friend whose child has ASD," or "I was watching a documentary on a child with Autism." It is even in our entertainment with movies such as *Temple Grandin* and television shows like *Atypical*. Although awareness of Autism is prevalent, understanding it has yet to be captured.

My colleagues and I have a saying, "If you've met one child with Autism, you've met one child with Autism." This is what drives most of us who have chosen this area of psychology to remain in this area. Children who are on the spectrum are a gift, an anomaly, but a gift nonetheless. Alli has done a masterful job capturing this in her book. It is an honest look at the beauty and challenges that children, parents, and families of kids with ASD all face.

What I most appreciate is how Alli walks the reader through the very common "stages" of accepting what ASD means to her family. It's a roadmap for other parents facing a similar journey. She starts by addressing the elephant in the room—what to do once you have a diagnosis, and how to process the ever-evolving feelings that accompany this new reality. Bold advice is offered throughout the book, like not always just accepting what a doctor or expert says, but rather empowering parents to find answers and solutions that feel true to their child and beliefs.

Alli describes the many roadblocks she faced and continues to face as Caden grows up and his needs change. Like many parents, she tried the trends and fads and grasped for any intervention that showed potential to reduce the impact of interfering symptoms without losing her son. She shared the disappointment she experienced each time the latest attempt did not yield the results she had hoped for.

By addressing her failed attempts, Alli normalizes this experience for other parents and encourages them to allow forgiveness of themselves and to continue the search for what is right for their child. She emphasizes the importance of mothers not only taking care of their Autistic child, but also finding ways to remain present for their other children and for themselves.

Oftentimes, the focus is solely on the child who is on the spectrum. Alli tackles the issue of the family's need to accept and cope with the diagnosis head on. She acknowledges the challenges she has faced with dividing her minimal time amongst all three of her children, each of whom comes with his own unique set of needs, as well as making time to be a wife and an individual person.

Although awareness and acceptance are becoming more widespread, it takes those brave enough, like Alli, to share their unique story to help society understand the complexity and splendor of Autism. Her very real account of her own personal journey through stages of feeling broken to realize she, her family, and most important her son are not broken. The humor and hope she brings to a typically serious and dismal topic is refreshing.

I have been fortunate to have a long-standing working relationship with Alli and her family. I have personally worked with each of her beautiful boys, and been touched by the wonder that is Caden. I still remember him sauntering into my office for the first time, wearing shorts and a T-shirt with a winter hat on. He made no apologies or excuses for who he was; yet I was gifted to experience his honesty, humor, and take on life. As a professional, I read this book and see the application of research and advances in medicine and treatment to a real life story. As a parent, one can read this book and see the community of others out there, like Alli, who share a similar story, one filled with ups and downs, but a beautiful tale of how to help themselves and others see that their Autistic child is not broken.

DR. KAYCIE DEANE *is a psychologist in California. She earned her PhD from the University of California, Los Angeles, where she focused her graduate studies and research on the treatment of Autism Spectrum Disorder. During her training, she had access to leading researchers and groundbreaking research conducted through the UCLA Center for Autism Research and Treatment and collaborations with other universities. Since completing her doctorate, she has been in private practice, offering psychotherapy and assessments to diagnose Autism.*

ACKNOWLEDGMENTS

If I were to acknowledge everyone who has got me to where I am today, or supported me on this journey, I could write an entire second book. Every single person I have come in contact with has enriched my life in one way or another. There is no way to thank you all, but know that each one of you was in my heart as I wrote this book and shared the stories of my life.

To my **family**, you have been my constant support system, there for me every single day and the reason I kept going every time I thought I couldn't. I thank you.

To my **Mom friends**, you know who you are. Without your endless support, nights out for drinks, laughter and tears, I would not be the same mom I am today. You have listened to me have my moments of complaining and have shared in so many triumphs, always cheerleading me every step of the way. I guess I should really thank our kids for bringing us together, and I thank you for sticking with me.

To my **"Ride or Dies,"** the ones who are more like sisters, who call me out on my shit and don't need a badge to know where they stand in my life. You know me better than most. During the times I need to be picked up off the floor, you are always there even when I tell you I'm OK. You see and love me for who I am, flaws and all, and will always support me in all my craziness.

To my **high school friends**, my girls—Sweet Gals from '95—I love you. You know how much I cherish our friendships. Each one of you holds a special place in my heart. What an amazing thing we have. When we get together, it is like coming home, I can curl up on the couch and cry or dance as if no one is watching, and all of you would be right there with me.

To my **Soul Sisters** and teachers, the ones who have helped guide me through this journey. You have shown me new paths and ways of seeing the world around me. You have taught me to let go of my control and really see myself for the amazing mom and person I am. You have taught me to acknowledge my struggles and embrace them, no longer allowing them to control me. And most important, you have shown me how strong I am and that there is beauty in being vulnerable.

My new **Mom friends** at Renaissance—thank you for being in the thick of it with me and having daily conversations that are REAL.

ACKNOWLEDGMENTS

Velcro Shoes Moms: To all the moms and women who have allowed me to hold space for them, be the ear and shoulder they need while they have shared their stories with me, I am humbled and honored. Thank you for being so beautifully vulnerable and trusting me with your truths. You have all enriched my life more than you know and have allowed me to feel connected and not alone. We are in this together.

All the old school **21st Street Crew** who have always supported Tome. Dads struggle, too! You are always there with an early morning text or hundred, with check em's or something that couldn't wait another minute to share. The heckles and laughs that go on sometimes for days, and the endless friendships that have been since childhood. You have all meant the world to Tome (and me). Never judging, always up for a good time, and accepting him and us always.

Da Boys—you know who you are. Tome would not have gotten through this without friends like you to distract him with a good time, surf sesh, volleyball beating, and all the laughter and good times. I thank and love you all.

To all the people who believed in this project and put endless hours into helping me bring it to life, I thank you. **Stephanie Byers**, you helped me get this off my computer and through its first edits. Meeting by chance via the web and then realizing our children were at the same magical school, it was no coincidence you were a part of this journey. **Sharon Castlen**, you have been a gift, guiding me along the way, keeping me in check and always making sure that my voice was not lost. **Shannon**, you have been a support from the beginning, and your creativity and experience with an eye for design have been a blessing. **Lisa**, your belief in not only this project, but my story and life has kept me going at times. Thank you for your endless hours of editing and editing and editing again. And **Terry Nathan**, who happens to be my brother-in-law, thank you for all your connections through the Independent Book Publishers Association. Thank you for helping me get this book out to the world to be seen and heard. To **Jan Nathan**, my late mother-in-law and the founder of IBPA (formerly PMA), I hope you are proud. I think of you often as I write and feel your energy with me.

I would not have had anyone else capture the photo for the cover of my book. **Liz Lonky**, owner of Life Iz Photography, has been a part of my life and my kids' life since their birth. Literally, since birth. She was in the operating room with me as I had my C-sections and has captured my children through the years as they have grown. She SEES them, and the photo on this book cover embraces everything I wanted it to.

ENERGY MUSE—Timmi and Heather, I can't thank you enough. You played such a huge role at a pivotal place in my life. You made me look in the mirror and start becoming aware of the energy around me and the gifts that I have been given. You allowed me to open up and start to feel.

ACKNOWLEDGMENTS

Critters. Tome. Kyle. Caden. Maguire. Mom. Dad. Jenny. Shawn. Aaron. Wendy. Lindsay. Sara. Tricia. Cara Ryan Jake and Drew. Kim. Giuliana. Christine the Fairy Godmother. Erin. Chelsea. Kelly. Darri. Lisa. Melissa and Sweet Bradley. Paige. Jen Fox Rocks. Hillary. Lauren. Mia. Megan. Sara Kranz Schultz. Kari Keating. Katie Spooner. Eliana Moon. Corinne. Ashun. New Best Friend Jennifer. Roomie Jenn. Kristen. Harper. Dylan. Gavin O. Gavin K. and Sweet Juliet. Laura Moyer. Moriah. Monica Fyfe. Catherine. Kaycie Deane. Elizabeth Maynard. Heather Tuttle. Miss Tiffany. Mrs. Opfer. Mrs. Sokol. Mrs. Legaspie. Mrs. Cindy. Mrs. Whitt. Melanie West. Wendy Zopel. Mrs. Ruth. Mrs. Estella. First Steps for Kids. Angela Elliott Wingard. Miss Barbie. Annie and Ronnie. Ride to Fly. Ms. Terri. Mr. Purdy. Miss Berry. Mr. Maher. Miss Sherese. Mrs. A. J. Mrs. Oduro. Mr. Thomas. Ruby. Christina Morse. Nancy Pants. Mr. Barakat. Alexis Casillas. Carl Dickson. Chris Stretch. Pegs and Megs. Adrian Hall. Patty, David, and Christian. Nick Cote. Heather and Timmi. Deanna. Suzy Parker. Ann Frohoff. Corinne Rushing. Liz Lonky. Mr. Arnnold. Alyce Marie. Mr. Awesome. Bre, Cb, Kasto, Chio, Godfather Druie. Bob and Vesna. Surfers Healing. Best Day Foundation. Shanden and Kim. Surfing with Nixon. Camp Surf. Beach Camp. Chavez for Charity. Different Is Awesome. Jessica Patay. Dr. Julie Douglass and Janelle Holden. Muktha. Lauren Pressey. Scharffenberger. Chandra and Trilogy Spa. Allyn and Justin. Jessica Lococo. Renee Love.

MY THREE SONS

Today I am present. I sit and reflect on my journey that has brought me to where I am today. I am grateful and humble and passionate and full of love. I have opened up and am willing to receive the greatness that surrounds me. Amazing things happen when you allow them to. I believe there is greatness waiting for us all. My eyes are wide open, I see the world, beautiful and rich with color. My heart is full, and I am no longer searching for something greater—all I need, I have. My life is perfect today. My imperfections make me who I am and have empowered me to be a better wife and mother.

My three boys have been gifts, greater than I ever expected. Through all our struggles and triumphs, watching my boys discovering the world, I have found myself, and I am learning to be the best version of me. I would have never guessed my kids would be the ones teaching me.

KYLE

My sweet old soul. You have no idea how beautiful you are, both inside and out. Your heart is your gift. It is pure and innocent with the ability to touch my soul. You make me smile every day when you tell me you love me. I thought that was my job.

CADEN

My brown-eyed baby. You have taught me patience and kindness and to look at the world with colored glasses. There is beauty in everything, it is around us every day. You have taught me that we all have gifts, some for all to see and some to be shared with the ones we choose. You surprise me every day with your strength and have shown me that anything is possible.

MAGUIRE

My uniquely awesome sidekick. You know who you are and aren't afraid to let others see your colors. You light up the world with your charisma and charm and have been the sparkplug in our family. You're wise beyond your years, and nothing is unattainable when you want it. You may be the youngest in age, but most of the time, you are the big brother. The compassion you show and the love you have for your brothers bring me tears of happiness. Watching you cry when you are proud of them, or get angry and protect them when they are being teased—you are one cool little bro.

The mom that I dreamed of being when I was younger may not be who I am today… but I am so much more, and I wouldn't change one minute. So, thank you, boys, for allowing me to be your mom, flaws and all. Thank you for loving me and always telling me I am the best mom, even when I lose my patience. Thank you for teaching me the important things in life are right in front of me, and that all I ever need is my family. Thank you for your daily hugs, I love you and your smiling dimples that get me through each and every day. I LOVE YOU.

INTRODUCTION

THE JOURNEY

Life is tough. It is a journey filled with bumps and turns, but it is our journey to embrace and live. This book is a glimpse into my world as a mom with a son who has Autism and another who has a specific learning disorder. I will share with you my journey and what I have learned through tears and laughter.

I want to be the best mom I can. I want to be the best version of me. I admit that I struggle with judgment, distraction, lack of boundaries, and confidence at times, not to mention anxiety, stress, and with finding a space for calm in my life. Does this sound familiar to you?

Having kids in general is a blessing, a gift that most parents cherish. Having kids is also a job that is unguidable, unteachable, and unimaginably difficult. Being a parent to a kid or kids who need extra love and support, understanding and empathy, advocacy and strength, can leave any parent depleted—of energy, of time for oneself, even depleted of purpose. And alone.

Try to take some time to slow down and just be. Allow yourself to sit with your feelings and FEEL. As moms, we take on the world. We tend to stay busy and don't recognize all that we have on our plates. This is so important. So take a minute and acknowledge all you have done for your child, and how far you have come. Acknowledge the hardships you face, the difficult times. When these feelings arise, it's OK to give them space, it's OK to have a "shitty day," or throw yourself a pity party. *Just don't stay there.* Not acknowledging your feelings is where we get into trouble. Pretending everything's OK, that you have it all together, and your life is perfect—that's when disaster strikes. Pushing down your feelings will only come to bite you in the ass later. Trust me, I know.

For me, this journey started with my middle son, Caden. Early on, my own lack of understanding about Caden's Autism, plus constantly feeling judged by the world around me and not knowing where I fit in, made me feel like others saw my son as a problem—disabled, damaged, broken. I wish I had been armed back then with all that I know now. I would have been empowered to better support him and protect him from the world.

INTRODUCTION

Being a parent to a kid or kids who need extra love and support, understanding and empathy, advocacy and strength, can leave any parent depleted—of energy, of time for oneself, even depleted of purpose. And alone.

Caden appears normal, like any other "typical" kid. His behaviors are what made people stare, his behaviors are what made people judge. What was wrong with my Caden, who got so overly energetic being in a huge ball pit at a My Gym Children's Fitness Center that he would chomp down on one of the plastic balls? *Nothing.* Nothing was wrong with him. He was so excited and, I didn't know, experiencing sensory overload. Biting down on the ball was a release for him.

What was wrong with my Caden, who couldn't sit still or sat slouched in his chair? Aren't boys wild and crazy and restless? However, this, too, is a sensory-processing issue that prevents the body from feeling gravity's pull. In turn, his brain doesn't tell his muscles to sit up.

The brain controls what we think and feel, how we learn and remember, and the way we move and talk. But it also controls things we're less aware of—like the beating of our hearts and the digestion of our food.

Our brain is like a computer and is in control of our bodies. Our nervous system is the runner of information, relaying messages back and forth from the brain to different parts of the body.

When a message comes into the brain from anywhere in the body, the brain tells the body how to react. For example, if you touch a hot stove, the nerves in your skin shoot a message of pain to your brain. The brain then sends a message back telling the muscles in your hand to pull away. Luckily, this neurological relay race happens in an instant.

What was wrong with my Caden who stared at television for hours? What was wrong with my kid who paced back and forth along the fence during school recess? Again, *nothing was wrong, it was just Caden being Caden.*

HOWEVER, OUR JUDGMENTAL WORLD, WHICH HAS LITTLE KNOWLEDGE ABOUT KIDS WITH SPECIAL NEEDS, SEES KIDS LIKE CADEN AS BROKEN.

We all deal with our child's diagnosis in our own ways. Just like parenting in general, we do whatever we need to do to get through the day or the moment. Some of us grieve, mourning, as if we lost a child we never had. Others are terrified, not knowing what to do, and some of us are in disbelief, maybe even denial that anything could be "wrong" with our perfect child. However we deal as moms, there is no right or wrong. We have

INTRODUCTION

to wrap our heads around the diagnosis and feel strong in our beliefs and in our love for our child. We have to be strong to brave the storm and judgment we are about to face from the society that will only see the label. Never fear, because you are about to be amazed and forever changed by your child and his or her label, and you will soon learn, your child is far from broken.

THEY. ARE. NOT. BROKEN.

I am here to tell you: They. Are. Not. Broken. That is the most important lesson of this journey, and there have been many, many lessons. Gifts, really.

Among these gifts: I have learned that I need to forgive myself, work on myself, love myself, and give myself the time I need to heal.

We live in a big world, and we can very easily feel isolated, but *we are not alone*. Connecting with others is the most empowering feeling. In the process of connecting with parents around the world, I have learned and listened, shared and cried, and I have felt empathy when I needed it most. I have learned to embrace my kids for who they are and to recognize their gifts and talents within. I have learned to help them, not cure them. I have discovered, through trial and error, what can enhance their lives—including supplements and oils, tinctures and alternative medicines.

I move a million miles a minute and hardly ever sit still. If I actually stop, I often think I will not be able to get going again. My tough exterior may look all put together, but inside, I am vulnerable with tears that need to be shed. However, my fear is that, if I start crying, I probably won't be able to stop, so my eyes stay dry and my heart remains heavy at times. I began to write for me. It was therapeutic and a way to get my feelings out, so I could start to feel. Now, I write for parents who have kids with special needs and for parents who have kids who are unique and different. They are presents waiting to be unwrapped, in essence, gifts to discover. We all have our struggles, from tantrums in the car because our toddlers want to buckle their own seat belt, to extremely hard days with epileptic seizures. Connection can be powerful, and when moms come together, we are unstoppable.

> **CONNECTION CAN BE POWERFUL, AND WHEN MOMS COME TOGETHER, WE ARE UNSTOPPABLE.**

Connect yourself with others! There are so many amazing groups out there that can support you. Trying to navigate this special needs journey alone can be scary and it can be overwhelming. You need to find support with those who understand what you are going through. Sometimes we need to vent, be heard, sometimes we will be asked for advice or to listen, and sometimes we need a glass of wine and time with a friend.

As I take you through my journey, I want you to remember that your child is not broken. Life is not over or ruined, worse or damaged because of your child. It

INTRODUCTION

is the exact opposite. Your life is filled with wonder and discovery, it is filled with hope and love, and it is filled with gifts. You will learn to live your life as an "Autism Mom" (or Dad), and you will learn that your life doesn't need to be fixed—it is already perfect.

My journey is far from over and definitely not where I want it to be. There are things that I am working on and will continue to work on for the rest of my life. But for today, my life is complete. I am learning to love myself today. I am learning to believe in myself and put positive energy out to the world. I still don't know what my future holds, and I still have to trust and have faith, but I believe in my heart I am on the right path and am so grateful each and every day—grateful that this journey led me to create a place to share, a place to feel connected, and a place to be vulnerable and real.

I am now becoming the mom that I always dreamed of. I am living in the town where I grew up and raising three special boys. To say that I have been through a lot is an understatement, especially discovering that two of my three sons have learning difficulties. I have traveled and journeyed, shared and listened to so many stories from women living similar lives. Stories that have made me laugh and cry, stories that have made me feel grateful and empathetic, but all stories that have enriched my life.

ONE

MOM IDENTITY

Growing up, all I ever wanted was to be a mom. I dreamed about the day when I would have my own babies, and playing family would be my reality.

My husband, Tome—my best friend and the love of my life—gave me the gift of three beautiful sons, Kyle, Caden, and Maguire. I am in awe every day how these brothers can be so different, each with his unique gifts to share with the world. I will never stop asking, "How did I get so lucky to be their mom?"

But this was not my reality in the beginning. Instead, the difficulty of being a mom—being a *parent*—was like a slap in the face. I found myself overwhelmed and barely functioning on autopilot. I was running faster and doing more, but none of what I was doing was for me. There was no down time, no chance to catch my breath, no recharging my own batteries.

My visions of motherhood when I was a little girl did not look anything like the woman I was becoming. The mom version I'd become had turned me into someone I didn't want to be. It broke my heart.

Learning how to let go of what I hoped my life was going to be, was one of the most difficult things I have had to do. I still struggle with it today. These are not just hopes and dreams I had of being a mom, but my hopes and dreams for my kids. What I have learned is that you cannot plan or control the unknown. For someone like me who has controlled every aspect of her life, this has been my biggest life challenge. However, with challenges there can be rewards. I have become a stronger more loving mom than I could have ever imagined as a young girl. And my boys, they have taught me that the only thing I need to hope for them is health and happiness and to support them with whatever dreams they have for themselves. To hope for something they do not want for themselves does not serve anyone.

And then, at age two, Caden was diagnosed with Autism.

How could this be? Well, sure, maybe his speech was coming along a little slowly, but I saw no big, red flag telling me there was a problem. In fact, I had watched, amazed, as Caden would listen to a new song and then push the buttons on my cell phone to emulate the music. And he was a rock star when it came to drag-and-drop games. He'd play for hours, passing level after level.

So what if he became so mesmerized by these games that he couldn't hear me call his name? So what if he became so overstimulated when he had all his stuffed animals around him that he would jump on them almost as if attacking his favorite friend to give them a hug. So what that he bounced in his Johnny Jumper for hours in the doorway and he would finally fall asleep mid bounce.

We were, however, concerned about how far behind he was talking, so we took him to a speech therapist. He made good progress, and then the therapist sat us down. "Go to the Regional Center," she said, "and make an appointment to get Caden tested." She never used the word *Autism*.

So we did. Caden attended two assessments, the first was in a small room and took maybe half an hour. Caden found a light switch and was repeatedly flipping it up and down. I remember we were asked, "Does he do that at home?"

I can remember thinking this was one of the most ridiculous tests ever. How could someone in a one hour span give kids a diagnosis that would be with them for the rest of their lives. Regional Centers are a double-edged sword. We need them to give us a diagnosis so the state can help fund services to help our kids, and guide us through the process (that is what is supposed to happen). They can also be difficult to work with, insensitive to our personal situations and just another thing we have to deal with. I learned through the years to just suck it up. What I will recommend to you and to everyone who receives a diagnosis, do not take one person's opinion. One person's opinion is one person's opinion. As your child develops and grows his or her behaviors and learning difficulties will change. So do yourself and your child a favor and find someone you connect with and trust and get your child tested with a professional outside of the school and Regional Center.

"No," I answered, "but our switches are too high for him to reach."

A month later, we received a report confirming that Caden had Autism.

Autism was not even on my radar. There was no one in my family who had it, no one I was close to. I was clueless. Even before we got the diagnosis, I started reaching out to friends and acquaintances with children who had Autism, and I also googled it. Every single person I talked with stressed the same point: The second you get the diagnosis, get your child into treatment. The earlier the treatment, the better the results.

I quickly learned that Autism covers a broad range of conditions. The word *Autism* itself is practically useless as a description. It is more accurately called Autism Spectrum Disorder, or ASD. The California Department of Developmental Services says: "Autism is a neurodevelopmental disorder characterized by impairments in social relating, language, and by the presence of repetitive and stereotyped behaviors." That still didn't tell me what I needed to know.

I was swept away by a feeling of sadness, not for me but for Caden: I didn't know what was in store for him, but I knew this was not going to be an easy road.

I can remember sitting in my closet one day hysterically crying. I literally sat in my closet with my face in my hands, tears streaming uncontrollably down my face. Moments like these have been few in my life. I can count them on one hand. I'd forever been strong, putting on a brave face, never sitting still, and always being the first one to help others. Now I realize much of it was to shield me from dealing with my own life.

I had been conditioned to believe over the years that crying was a sign of weakness. Worse, if I were to start the tears, the chances were great that I wouldn't be able to pick myself up. I didn't have time for that.

If the speech therapist had not referred us, I would probably have let things slide, and we might have waited another two years. You might think your child's pediatrician will pick up on possible issues, but they only see a child for maybe 15 minutes at a time. They can only do so much.

My life was about to become a whirlwind, never slowing down and always looking for the next thing that would help my kids succeed in life. But as I sat in my closet this time, these tears were different; these were tears of acknowledgment, of hope and belief. I was about to jump, about to do the thing that scared me the most, sharing myself and my journey with the world and learning to love myself through each step. These tears were telling me it was time... And so my journey began.

I was nearly forty years old. It was time to stop being afraid, to take a chance, to believe in myself and to follow an unfamiliar path. I had no idea where it would lead me. I knew that I wanted to stop living on a hamster wheel. Do you remember the movie *Groundhog Day* with Bill Murray? He lives the same day over and over, until he finally learns his lesson. That's how I was feeling.

I was living a very unpurposeful life, for me. Clearly, I served a purpose to my kids and my husband, but I had no passion and felt like there was something bigger out there that I was supposed to be doing. Lost and not sure where to look for answers, I decided to reach out to friends who are energy readers.

I found myself sitting in a room filled with every kind of crystal and stone, every shape, color, and size. They were beautiful. I shared my story and my reason for being there, and we began some exercises. I was instructed to choose the stones to which I was most drawn, as many as I wanted. I chose four stones:

- The Selenite Stone, which removes blocked energy, cleanses and protects

- The Amazonite Stone, which represents luck, hope, truth, and manifestation

- The Pyrite Stone, another stone for luck, wealth, and manifestation

- The Angelite Stone or Stone of the Angels, the properties of which are tranquility, healing, and connection to angels.

Next, I was instructed to select one card from each of seven stacks of Angel cards. I chose:

- Hello and Goodbye, which represents impending change to make things better.

- Apollo, which refers to focus on personal strengths.

- The Honeybee card, which translates into letting compassion and forgiveness be top priority.

- Clairsentience, or Archangel Raguel, which conveys a message to be conscious of your recurring physical and emotional feelings, as they signify divine guidance.

- The Smokey Quartz card represents grounding and stabilizing and brings centering energy.

- Next, the Mediumship card signifies the natural ability to connect with departed loved ones.

- Last, Giraffe Foresight means to be able to see what is in store for the future.

As I sat in this room feeling all the energy that surrounded me, I knew things were going to change. I knew I was going to start seeing what was in front of me and trusting in the path that lay ahead.

And that is exactly what happened.

The best thing I have done for myself is to ask for help. I was stuck, not knowing what to do with my life, but knowing I wasn't happy. I was sitting in a place of overwhelm and I was letting it consume me. Being overwhelmed can be paralyzing, and we end up doing nothing, we are frozen. So, we do what we know, which is getting back on our hamster wheel and running. Don't allow yourself to sit in overwhelm. Ask for help, do something, find some direction and get uncomfortable. If you want to change, you are going to need to do something different.

I began meditating every day, something I had never done before. The thought of sitting still in my own thoughts was beyond difficult for me, but I did it. Within this quiet time, learning more about myself, I decided to start writing, again something I had never done before. My writing turned into a place for me to share my thoughts and feelings, my stories, my life.

My writing transformed into a blog, which has opened so many doors. The people I have met have changed my life and are now part of my journey. With my eyes and heart open, I was seeing the world around me in a new light. I was listening to people and really hearing what they were saying. My quickness to judge others slowly turned into compassion and wanting to shout out, "You're different and it's *awesome*."

I found my path, even though I had no idea exactly where it would take me. Filled with bumps and curves, I am on it. I am doing what I do best, talking and connecting. I am sharing stories that I am not ashamed of, because they have created the story of my life. I am doing my best to be vulnerable and real and to tell my stories as they should be told. On this journey, I am slowly discovering who I am. I am not just a mom of three boys, or a mom of kids with special needs. I am all that, and so much more.

In the daily grind of being a mom, a wife, and maintaining a career, I had lost my spark, my sense of direction, my *self*. I had put all others before me, my needs taking the backseat as life passed me by. It is now my time to take care of myself. Without putting my family to the side, I am learning to simplify my life and focus on what is important. I am taking control of the things I've neglected and I have begun the work on me; my mind, body, and soul. I will follow my passion and learn to believe in myself—that I am worthy of the gifts I have been given.

> I AM LEARNING TO SIMPLIFY MY LIFE AND FOCUS ON WHAT IS IMPORTANT.

I needed to create a place for all these narratives to be shared, where moms can come and feel connected and not alone. I decided what was needed was a sisterhood of moms who have an unspoken understanding of one another, allowing us to support one another and give advice, or just listen. I do not have all the answers, but we are all in this together. This has not been an easy path, but it has been filled with color.

Light cannot shine without darkness. It is sometimes in our darkest moments we see the light. I was able to find myself when I thought my life couldn't get any worse. I was able to find my purpose and my WHY for getting up every morning and LIVING.

TWO

DAD CAN FIX IT

From Tome: The first time I tried to write my chapter about Caden, it was very matter of fact and just about the timeline of Caden's issues, diagnosis, and treatment. After writing it and then reading it, I realized two things that were not relayed in the first version. One, the chapter did not properly give enough credit for all the hard work that Caden did to transform into the person Caden was then and who he is today. Second, and more important, I did not give enough recognition and respect to my amazing wife, Alli, who has taken on all the responsibilities and pushed hard, momma bear hard, to fight for the rights of her child.

Alli's momma bear instincts kicked in big time, and she went to work researching and devoting most of her time finding out more information on what can be done to help a child with Autism. I have always been in awe of Alli's beauty, drive, and determination. But to see her put all her efforts into helping our son was inspiring. Alli reached out to all her friends and friends of friends for guidance, support, and information from anyone with a child on the spectrum. She talked to multiple companies to find the best one that could help and treat Caden. She researched Caden's rights to find out what the state and local districts were required to provide. Alli basically became Caden's champion because that's what a momma bear does for her cub but also to be able to help other parents and children who are affected by this affliction. You see, when I was first dating Alli, one of the best attributes that I recognized in her was that she was always willing to sacrifice her personal time to help her family and friends.

When we first got the news of Caden's diagnosis, I had so many thoughts and emotions running through my head. Will he ever be able to talk to us? Will he have some unbelievable counting and math skills like the character played by Dustin Hoffman in *Rain Man*? Will he be able to have a job or drive a car? What about a girlfriend? The unanswerable questions and the unknown future were too much to comprehend and at times were so overwhelming that I couldn't think or concentrate on anything. My brain was spinning out of control, trying to understand what my life and role as a father were now going to be like with a child with Autism. I had to sit back, close my eyes, and take deep breaths to refocus myself. As men and fathers, all we want to do is fix things. There were times when I would just hold Caden and rock back and forth while tears filled my eyes and slowly ran down my cheeks, knowing I couldn't "fix" this. I felt helpless.

> AS MEN AND FATHERS, ALL WE WANT TO DO IS FIX THINGS. I COULDN'T FIX THIS. I FELT HELPLESS.

Slowly, through the help of the ABA therapists, I got to see and understand more of Caden's personality and how to interact with him. I was finally able to build a relationship with Caden by playing certain games and engage with him using techniques the therapists used. I found out Caden likes music. I was surprised to see that Caden is funny and has a witty sense of humor. Caden's imagination was mesmerizing. There were so many instances that caught me by surprise because I had jumped to the conclusion that he was not going to be able to do things or interact in a way that I expected. The more I found out about Caden, the more I understood that Autism isn't the end of your relationship

> THE MORE I FOUND OUT ABOUT CADEN, THE MORE I UNDERSTOOD THAT AUTISM ISN'T THE END OF YOUR RELATIONSHIP WITH YOUR CHILD.

with your child. I was given a different door leading to a different hallway that looks through different windows that opened my eyes to a different way of looking at the world. And it is amazing!

Society has trained me to understand and view the world and the people around me from a "normal" perspective. Caden has shown me that certain people not only think outside the box but ARE outside the box, looking at the box from such a vastly different perspective it is possible to see the box as something entirely different. And it is OK to view it that way.

It has been an extremely tough road with twists and turns so sharp and unexpected that I was almost thrown off multiple times. We faced barriers that seemed impossible to get around. Caden would make huge strides and reach plateaus only to have setbacks. I felt like I was on the game "Chutes and Ladders," going forward and then sliding back down a level that would cause frustration and anger. The communication between Caden and I was the toughest. I needed information to be able to give my son what he wanted but to also form a relationship.

Caden worked hard every day, and as he would improve, I got better at understanding his special perspective. I started feeling proud of my son. We would work together toward a common goal and build a companionship. We had fun playing video games together. I laughed at his jokes and his sense of humor. I had a smile on my face instead of worry.

Caden would continue his hard work for many years, reaching many milestones, and getting better at socially interacting with us as his parents, his grandparents, and his brothers. To this day, Caden is the most compliant of all the boys. I believe he developed an understanding that all things will take some effort and that there will always be someone who is going to ask him to perform a chore, task, or instruction. Caden went on to elementary school and over the six years he was there, he formed friendships with other kids and those kids developed friendships with Caden. These friends didn't see Caden with a disability. They saw a funny, outgoing, and imaginative boy. These friends recognized Caden's weaknesses and aided him when he needed help. That is true friendship.

> **THESE FRIENDS DIDN'T SEE CADEN WITH A DISABILITY. THEY SAW A FUNNY, OUTGOING, AND IMAGINATIVE BOY.**

THREE

IT TAKES A VILLAGE

My world today would not be the same without my village. I have been so fortunate to have an absolutely remarkable husband, parents who wholeheartedly support me any way they can, friends who are always there for me with a moment's notice, and a team of therapists who have been a huge part of my life since 2011. These very important people are my village, and without them, I would not be who I am today, nor would my children. The biggest lesson I learned was to include them in my daily life and my challenges. I am the village chief, but my village lifts me up and gives me the strength and courage to get through the days, and I am forever grateful.

Understand this: We all have the ability to create a village. Yours may consist of your spouse or significant other, extended family members, and friends who might feel more like blood relatives. They are there for you, so utilize them.

> **WE ALL HAVE THE ABILITY TO CREATE A VILLAGE.**

Sometimes all you need is a sounding board or a shoulder to cry on. Other times, you need a relief pitcher or a clone of yourself because you can't be in two places at the same time.

Being a parent is one of the hardest but most pivotal jobs in the world. We shape lives, which means we are on the clock 24/7. What other job entails endless work with no pay? In all actuality, we pay our kids—in love and selfless time—as we slave, clean, prepare meals (some of us cook, but me, not so much), organize social activities, cheerlead at every sporting event, do homework (which even challenges me), are the hygiene police and, lest we forget, Uber/taxi drive them everywhere! The list is endless.

I love seeing the look on people's faces when they ask me how many kids I have. Their response: "You have three boys? Oh, honey, I'm so sorry." Why are they sorry? Because I don't have a girl? Or because they think my boys are little hellions? And why do people think they can just share their opinion with me anyway? Yes, my boys are a handful at times, but that is part of the beauty of being my specific version of a mom. My kids are my everything, and I embrace the good, the bad, and the ugly. They fill my life with color.

Don't you think it's amazing how much we do as moms? I guarantee not one of us dreamed of being a taxi driver as a little girl. Who knew?! According to Instagram, here is how to be a good mom in 2019:

Make sure your children's academic, emotional, psychological, mental, spiritual, physical, nutritional, and social needs are met while being careful not to overstimulate, underestimate, improperly medicate, helicopter, or neglect them in a screen-free, positive, socially conscious, egalitarian but also authoritative, nurturing but fostering independence, gentle but not overly permissive, pesticide-free, two-story, multilingual home preferably in a cul-de-sac with a backyard. Also don't forget the coconut oil. You got that, Mom?

All children are born with unique gifts, all wrapped up waiting to be discovered. My boys are special in their own ways, as are your kids. My older two, Kyle and Caden, are very similar, which makes sense because they both have learning difficulties. Maguire, the youngest, is one of a kind. While Kyle and Caden are computer-video-game-Lego kids who can lounge all day and prefer to be in their "comfort zone," Maguire needs to be doing something. He is my sports kid. As young as age eight, he was playing every team sport. Between Maguire's sports and all the therapy sessions for Kyle and Caden, I have become chauffeur extraordinaire.

Early on, Tome worked and I spent the day with therapists or researching the next program in which to enroll Caden. I attended all the meetings at school, IEPs, doctors' appointments, and social programs. I was the one who heard the feedback from the many specialists and took in the emotions, hearing about Caden's struggles and his progress. By the end of the day, when Tome came home from work or my mom called to see how my day had been, I was emotionally exhausted, and I rarely shared. Thus, by the end of the day, I could not retell what went on and if I did, the information would only be partial. The emotional drain of recalling everything was too much for me, so I just kept it to myself. After all, I was strong and I could handle it.

Or so I thought.

But no one can do this alone.

For one thing, when you attend any type of meeting, **NO ONE CAN DO THIS ALONE.** especially an IEP, your stress level, anxiety, and nerves are all heightened. Throw in emotion to the mix, and it can lead to disaster. This is why so many knowledgeable people recommend bringing an advocate or someone close to you when attending meetings. Parents often lose their train of thought or get so upset about a particular personal discovery that they zone out or can only focus on that one thing. They can forget to ask important questions and get off topic very easily. Having someone there to take notes or remind you of what needs to be accomplished in the meeting is vital.

I honestly do not know what I would do if I did not have my parents. When Caden was first diagnosed, I remember my mom asking if I had googled "Autism." I mean, that is like googling "cancer," isn't it? It's ubiquitous.

Knowing what I know now, I was really naive to think I could take this all on by myself. I thought I was doing my husband a favor. I knew he had to go to work and be present, and I didn't want to burden him with all the emotional exhaustion that came with these meetings. On top of that, I knew it was difficult for him to take off work, so I just didn't ask. Once you get the ball rolling, and you have taken this all on for yourself, it is hard to expect your partner to understand what you are going through. I didn't let my husband in and at the same time, I was desperate for help.

I have to remember that, when I was growing up, Autism wasn't a common diagnosis. We had "different" kids who attended my school, kids who couldn't sit still and behaved in ways no one understood. There was also a classroom dedicated to special needs students who were more severely challenged. But then, as kids ourselves, we just blew it off. It was what it was.

So when my parents learned Caden was Autistic, it was understandably foreign to them. In the beginning, it was sometimes lonely and overwhelming for me. I felt the weight of the world on my shoulders.

I found myself at times drowning in all the daily-life things I had to do plus this new journey of exploration to help Caden. That's when Papa (my dad) stepped in to share my chauffeur duties.

Papa is one of the most extraordinary people I know. He does everything for everyone always and never expects anything in return. He is the epitome of a Nice Guy. He is the one everyone wants to talk to and hang out with; the person you want to be your best friend.

How blessed I am to have him as my dad. He is a huge part of my life and my boys' lives. He has been there since the day they were each born and sees them almost every day. It fills my heart with so much joy to know that my boys will have cherished memories of their Papa. Papa takes the boys on adventures, bike riding, playing at the boulders by the beach (their favorite), on his boat, vacations of all kinds, to the movies, or just running errands with him to spend time and hang out.

IT TAKES A VILLAGE

My boys never turn down Papa. For one thing, they know a shave ice will be part of the deal. I can say with certainty that I would not have been able to do what I did or be the mom I am without my dad. He takes at least one shift a day to drop off or pick up one kid to a sports practice or therapy session, so I don't have to run around like a chicken with my head cut off (which I do anyways). He is always there to help.

Nana is my marvelous mother. Nana loves the boys as if they were her own. She spoils them and, bless her heart, listens to Kyle as he shares every single Lego creation he has made (it takes an hour every time). She spent her life working so that she could provide the best life for all of us. We all give her a hard time for being a workaholic, but the truth is, if she didn't work, my kids wouldn't be in all the life-saving therapies they need, or the sports programs or special classes. She is the biggest warrior in my village.

> "ALONE WE CAN DO SO LITTLE; TOGETHER WE CAN DO SO MUCH."
> —HELEN KELLER

Nana and I are both learning together that work and money aren't the most important things in life. What's most important is, of course, family. We remind each other to enjoy every day and be grateful and be aware that we are blessed. I do not know what I would do without my close relationship with my mom. She is my best friend and my go-to person. She also had three children—I am the middle child, sandwiched by two brothers. Perhaps that partly explains our closeness, our mother/daughter bond.

However, there are times when she admittedly doesn't understand my world or what I go through. Nevertheless, she is empathetic and always there for me. She never judges my parenting and is my biggest cheerleader. My mom tells me that she thinks I am an incredible mother, and every day she is in awe of me. Those words will stay with me forever. It is the greatest compliment, coming from someone I love and admire so much.

My friends keep me sane on a daily basis. They are the people I check in with each day. They listen and support me, and they trust in me to share their daily triumphs and struggles. Even though the majority of my friends do not have kids with special needs, they do have kids, and they understand motherhood is a hard job. They are the ones I call on to vent or get a much needed cocktail, and they will always be there for me with unconditional love and no judgment. Every once in a while, I get stopped in my tracks with someone giving me a compliment. I am not good at accepting praise. It makes me very

> **BE STRONG ENOUGH TO STAND ALONE, SMART ENOUGH TO KNOW WHEN YOU NEED HELP, AND BRAVE ENOUGH TO ASK FOR IT.**

uncomfortable, but I am trying to learn to just say "thank you."

I have been told: "I don't know how you do it. You have so much on your plate, three boys, a career, and all the things you do for Caden, and you never complain. You are amazing!" It is very easy to look at someone's life from the outside. I don't see what my friends see in me. I do what I need to do. I simply have had no other choice.

And, of course, I cannot forget to give a shout out to all the teachers who have worked so closely with Caden, especially the one and only Miss Tiffany! She was my son's aide, who came into our lives and embraced Caden, pushing him to find his inner self. She gave Caden a safe place to discover and be Caden.

Also there's his special education teacher, who saw all the greatness and potential inside and didn't allow him to settle. To all the occupational therapists, speech therapists, neuropsychologists, educational therapists, doctors, and dentists who have worked with us through the years, I thank you. The ABA therapists who spent endless hours at our house for six years, I appreciate you. All these selfless caregivers have become a part of our family, and they probably saw more of me than they wanted.

And most important, the man who stole my heart with his kind soul and makes me feel special every day—my sidekick, partner in crime, and very best friend, my husband, Tome. Without him, I simply would not be.

I am so grateful for his belief in me, allowing me to take the reins in doing what's needed for our children and their disabilities. He heads off to work every day to crunch numbers and pay our stack of doctors' and therapy bills, allowing me to be home with the kids, which has permitted them to flourish.

He trusts me to make decisions and is my sounding board for advice. He has never once questioned or doubted any decision I have made. He acknowledges that meetings, therapists, talking with teachers, and knowing every aspect of our kids' lives comprise my full-time job.

Tome deals with my exhaustion and, although he hasn't actually experienced a day in my life, he is compassionate and understanding. He is the only other person in this world who loves our kids as much as I do. He is there to lean on and to hold me, that is, if he can slow me down long enough to grab me.

The days I need to burst into tears and have a full-on breakdown, he is the one who picks me up. I thank God every day for him. He is my soul mate in every sense, and we were given these exceptional kids for a reason.

Relationships are hard, no doubt. The challenges of being a parent in a normal situation can be stressful and results in marriages crumbling. The financial strain this has put on our family at times seems unbearable.

However, we have made it through the toughest of these times and love each other more every single day, even on the days when we need a break from each other. I am proud of our strength as a couple, and I know that we are the driving force in helping our kids be the best versions of themselves.

All these people are my village. Without my village, my life would be one I wouldn't want to live. Caden would not be where he is—I can't imagine what he would be like today without all the therapy and programs he has gone through. And I am certain I would not be who I am today. I would not be the proud mother of three amazing boys. I would not be able to see all the greatness in Caden as he prepares to spread his wings and soar. I would not be able to see how rich and colorful my life is.

It is my village that has allowed me to open my eyes and see. I am grateful every day for being allowed to be Caden's mom. Instead of a life that could have been boring, bland, and grey, leaving nothing to the imagination, I have learned to be compassionate and kind, patient and accepting.

> CADEN HAS TAUGHT ME TO LOOK WITHIN AND DISCOVER WHO I AM.

Caden has taught me to look within and discover who I am. He teaches me every day about the beauty in people and the gifts they have to offer. I have been blessed with the gift of Caden and his Autism.

FOUR

A GIFT OF EMPOWERMENT

"My goal is to have Caden mainstreamed by kindergarten."

Caden was three years old the first time I made that statement. He was starting preschool when we had his initial IEP meeting. Caden had only been diagnosed with Autism a year earlier, and it had been a whirlwind of a year.

I couldn't help thinking that this happy little boy, with a world of opportunities at his fingertips, wouldn't have the same opportunities as other children. Because mainstreaming was the perceived or normal benchmark, that became my target.

You may be asking what, exactly, does it mean to mainstream a child? Put simply, in education it means nothing more than moving a child out of special education, self-contained classrooms and into regular classrooms—the "mainstream" of schooling. This stemmed from Public Law 94-142, passed by Congress in 1975, requiring that all children be educated in "the least restrictive environment."

The Condition of Education 2018, published by the Department of Education, reports that the number of students ages three to twenty-one who are receiving special education services increased from 6.6 million to 6.7 million from the 2014–15 school year to the 2015–16 school year. This comprises about 13 percent of all students. The take-away here is that the number of children diagnosed with so-called learning disabilities is on the rise.

So, that was my original goal, to have Caden mainstreamed by kindergarten. Then, at his last IEP meeting before his transition to elementary school, I was asked what my goals were for him. I laughed for, oh, so many reasons.

Once you accept that your child will be different, not better or worse—just different—that's the first step.

Up to this point, I had learned a great deal about Caden—his gifts and his diagnosis—and I had learned a lot about me. I laughed because the year before, I didn't know anything and I was panicked. I was also both hopeful and scared of what the future might hold and what it would look like for my baby. This IEP meeting was different, because I was sitting as a proud mama. Caden had been working eight hours a day, six

MAINSTREAM VS. INCLUSION

"Love me as I am. Don't make me feel less than I am. I don't need to fit into your idea of perfect to be imperfectly great."

I wish I knew then what I know now. I wish I was as strong as I am now. I always believed in Caden and never once doubted his abilities, but I wish I didn't want something for him that he didn't want for himself or he wasn't ready to embrace. I wasn't seeing what was right in front of me, I was worried about what others were seeing, what others might be thinking. I was trying to make Caden blend in, when he was meant to stand out. I am grateful that our society is learning the importance of inclusivity and schools are implementing it into their classrooms.

"Inclusive education is about embracing all, making a commitment to do whatever it takes to provide each student in the community an inalienable right to belong, not be excluded. Inclusion assumes that living and learning together is a better way that benefits everyone, not just children who are labeled as having a difference" (Falvey, Givner & Kimm, 1995, p. 8). —Thinkinclusiv.us days a week. All Caden knows is to work, that is his life. He doesn't know any other way.

He overcame obstacles that were so difficult for him and, as frustrated as he would sometimes get, he never gave up. Holding a pencil correctly, making eye contact, saying "hi" to even his mom and dad, sharing, taking turns, learning not to get up and wander when he wasn't supposed to, interacting with peers, using scissors, and responding when his name was called—these were all major accomplishments, and I was beyond proud.

> "IF YOU ARE ALWAYS TRYING TO BE NORMAL, YOU WILL NEVER KNOW HOW AMAZING YOU CAN BE."
>
> —MAYA ANGELOU

There were so many reasons my heart was filled with joy at that meeting, and that brought tears to my eyes. Parents often discuss the negative of what their child can't do, but if they take a moment to reflect, they will realize their kid is a *rock star*!

That was the moment when I understood my goal had changed. My new goal was for Caden to simply be happy. Happy and healthy. I wanted and I still want for my son to be happy, healthy, and not to struggle through life.

I was reminded recently by a mom whose two-year-old was just diagnosed that it doesn't help to look forward, because we have no control over the future. We need to take each day as it comes, and do

A GIFT OF EMPOWERMENT

"It shouldn't matter how slowly a child learns. What matters is that we encourage them to never stop trying." —Robert John Meehan

Celebrate all the small things. It can be difficult to understand how something that can come so easy for us, can be extremely difficult for our kids. We don't see the complexities of how our brain works and communicates with the rest of our body. Celebrate when your kid learns to hop, or snap their fingers (this one is still difficult for Caden). Make a big deal when they use their pencil correctly or come out of the bathroom with their pants not twisted. Let your child see how proud you are of them, for their accomplishments and for who they are. Don't compare them to your other children, which can be easy to do, and don't ever let them feel less than.

the best we can to help our kids in the moment. For parents new to this journey, remember this: You will receive much advice and many words of wisdom, but as parents, we are the ones who know our children best. We are going to be their advocates, and we will know what they need better than anyone else. Whatever diagnoses and labels we are handed, whatever they may be, take them as a gifts and do something positive with them. We can be empowered by a diagnosis—it gives us a starting point and a way to measure our journey.

Diagnosis or not, your kid is who he/she is. Five minutes before you received his or her diagnosis, your child was the same person as now. So why all of a sudden treat your child differently? Your love for your child hasn't changed. In life, all we want to do is help our children be the best they can be. Now, with a diagnosis, you can! You now have direction, you now have some answers and you now have understanding.

Before Caden was diagnosed, I remember being at the Regional Center when a therapist asked, "Why is your son playing with the light switch, flipping it on and off?" I bristled, thinking, "Well, if the light switch was higher than two feet from the floor, my son would probably not be interested. And what the hell do you know anyway? You were only with my kid for an hour and you think you can tell me about my son? You know *nothing* about my son!"

My blood boiled as we left our assessment at the Regional Center. I held Caden tight and close to my body like I was fleeing wolves. I was the mama bear protecting my cub.

We received the Autism diagnosis a month later, and I honestly don't even remember opening the letter or reading the words. I already knew that Caden needed help and, diagnosis or not, I would do whatever needed to be done. I learned real quick that the diagnosis was a gift, because it gave me power to seek out therapies that would be invaluable to Caden's future success.

Accepting the Autism diagnosis was not something I ever questioned. It was what it was. Since day one, I always looked at it as information. Caden was the same adorable, big-brown-eyed, dimpled, smiley toddler he had been before the diagnosis. Nothing had changed except that I now had this information, this gift that I could choose to use as I wanted. We were fortunate to have close friends with a son who was also Autistic, and they urged us not to wait one day, that early intervention is the key to closing the gap.

We started ABA therapy the very next week. Caden would stand at the door in the morning in his diaper, bottle hanging from his mouth. The first session lasted from 8:30 a.m. until noon, and then the second round was from 12:30 until 4:00 p.m. It was a full-time gig.

Applied Behavior Analysis focuses on developing procedures that will produce observable changes in behavior and uses both operant conditioning and classical conditioning techniques.

At this time I had Kyle, my oldest who was just four, and I was pregnant with my third son. I was a robot, on autopilot at best; multitasking at its most intense. I did not have a minute to slow down, to stop, take a breath, think, or feel sorry for myself or my family. It took years before I shed a tear. I accepted Caden's diagnosis, and I immersed myself in making him my priority.

> **IT TOOK YEARS BEFORE I SHED A TEAR.**

In high school, my friends and I would joke that "Cliff" was one of our best friends. I hated reading, so Cliff Notes were the only way I survived English classes. There is no doubt that I probably have some sort of attention deficit hyperactivity disorder myself, because reading for me is torture. It would take me forever to read one page, and when I did, I had no idea what I had just read. But when it came to learning about Autism, I couldn't seem to find any Cliff Notes on the subject.

I found a book that was written by a celebrity, about her son having Autism. She was funny and I thought it would be an easy read for me. I read it aloud to my husband as we traveled by car on vacation. "This book sucks!" I told him. It was depressing and gave me little hope for my son's future. I sat and thought, Caden is never going to do well in school, never have friends, or a girlfriend, never play sports or be in a play, never go to college or have a job…. He was two! I was just beginning this journey, I needed to believe that my son was going to be OK. That was my first and last attempt to find a book to educate and console me.

About six months after Caden's diagnosis, we were knee deep in therapy and looking at other resources for him. At a mandatory meeting at the Regional Center, Tome and I sat next to each other. There were twelve chairs that created a circle, and five other couples joined us. The looks on their faces ranged from petrified, to hopeless, to scared, anxious, and sad, and looking at them made me very uneasy. We had to go around the room, introduce ourselves, and talk about our child in as much detail as we felt comfortable with. Tome and I were last to speak.

IT'S OK TO ASK FOR HELP.

As these parents started to share their experiences, tears streamed down their faces. Most of these families had just been given the diagnosis of their son or daughter a week prior and had not yet had the chance to digest the news. Their stories were heartbreaking, and I just wanted to get up and give them all a hug.

One dad said that his toddler was self-harming. He would hit his head so hard against the wall that they had to have him start wearing a helmet. He would bite and scratch his arms until they bled.

Another mom talked about her daughter who would lick the walls outside their house. She was vitamin deficient, and they were having a hard time getting her to eat anything. At the time, they were force feeding her nutrition drinks. These parents sounded empty, at a loss, and definitely hopeless. When it was our turn to talk about Caden, I was nervous. Remember, I constantly felt judged by parents everywhere I took Caden. Looks of confusion and wondering what was "wrong" with him. Now I was in an area where we were all sharing, a safe place, but I still felt vulnerable, like I was about to be judged.

We said Caden was a typical child for the most part, happy and always laughing, not many behaviors untypical for a two-year-old. He didn't have tantrums or outbursts or unusual ticks. To most people, he seemed typical. What he demonstrated was an overly focused mindset, times when we could not get his attention, and sensory overload—a toddler who liked to rock in his crib and bang his head against the headboard.

After listening to the other parents, I was embarrassed. Our challenges seemed insignificant in comparison. Nonetheless, our problems were still our problems, our obstacles to overcome. And the reality was that these problems were not insignificant—they were deep and complex, and we had no idea what lay ahead in our journey. Looking around the room, it was clear to me that none of these parents knew what to do.

> **THESE PROBLEMS WERE NOT INSIGNIFICANT—THEY WERE DEEP AND COMPLEX.**

They were in a state of shock and felt alone. Simply put, you don't know what you don't know.

I hesitantly shared how we had been in therapy with Caden for almost six months. Parents' faces began to lighten, and I realized I was giving them what they all craved—*hope*. They needed someone to tell them that their life wasn't over, that things would get better from here, that there were people like me, open and willing to share my story and help those who needed guidance. *They weren't alone.*

Surround yourself with people that will support you during this journey. The special needs community can be whatever you want it to be for you. It is large and powerful and very accessible. Don't ever settle, seek advice and always ask questions. Follow your motherly intuition, it is a real thing. You know your child better than anyone, don't ever let anyone make you second guess that.

Unfortunately, the system—that is, the resources and guidance available for families dealing with Autism—is wracked with bureaucratic rules and regulations. Honestly, what I used to say—and say frequently—was that "they prey on the stupid." Not the most eloquent choice of words, but true. The government, the schools, they rely on people not educating themselves and not advocating fiercely for their children. There is not going to be a knock on your door or a phone call from someone offering you everything you are missing out on. They aren't going to tell you all the services and options there are for your child that could be funded by the state. That is just not going to happen. If you don't get out there and fight and educate yourself, all the amazing things your child is supposed to share with the world will go unseen. Empower yourself with knowledge.

In this eight-year journey as a mom to a son with Autism, I am more proud than ever. I have embraced who my son is, and am seeing glimpses of color trying to burst out of his skin (that's how I think of his potential). He is getting ready to explode, like a piñata, sprinkling the world with surprises. I am in awe each and every day I learn more about Caden, and it is an overwhelming feeling to see him discover for himself who he is.

> **HE IS GETTING READY TO EXPLODE, LIKE A PIÑATA, SPRINKLING THE WORLD WITH SURPRISES.**

FIVE

I AM CADEN

Hi. My name is Caden and I am going to talk to you about how it is to be Autistic. It is not a bad thing, it is a gift from God. Sometimes I think that my Autism doesn't have any good, but it really does, in my heart and connecting to others.

I am a kid who has Autism, but it hasn't been that way my entire life. Or I didn't know about it my entire life. Probably before I was born, my mom took some really bad medicine, or vaccines that might have made me Autistic or something. My mom told me they don't know exactly what causes Autism, but it could be the vaccines I got as a baby, and all the bad stuff that is now killing our planet. When the doctor told

IT IS NOT A BAD THING, IT IS A GIFT FROM GOD.

my parents I had Autism, they were probably shocked about it.

When I was little, I wasn't able to be with others, not being able to connect with others, all because I had Autism. My life was very awful because I couldn't be with others. I thought I was different from others because I thought Autism was something bad. I thought it was like a virus or something, so I didn't play with others so they wouldn't get sick.

Mostly everything in my life has been hard, but I still do it. I felt sad and depressed in the past. When my mom first talked to me about this Autistic thing, I thought I was different. So I was mostly depressed. When I was young, I thought being different and having Autism was kind of like having a disease. But as I grew up, I learned it was something special. I am very special to have these Autistic powers.

> **I AM VERY SPECIAL TO HAVE THESE AUTISTIC POWERS.**

I am different from other kids. We don't always act different. Normal people go a straight way, and Autistic people go a different way. It's not bad to go a different way.

If I had to give someone advice on what it's like to have Autism, I would tell them all about my life with Autism and it would make them feel better.

One of the best things I like about me is that I am not the best artist, but I think I am and I love it. I love my fluffy cat, Cookie, even though he has fleas sometimes. I have a lot of friends, and I think people like me. I am funny, a little weird, and happy.

Having Autism isn't bad. It is nice to be me. I like people, I like video games, I get to go to school. I sometimes feel different though. I like things that not many people like. I think when I was at my elementary school, I was tagged as disabled, and that made me not want to play with people. It made me feel like no one wanted to play with me. I did play with people sometimes, but not that much. I am just different from all of them. They think I am weird. Sometimes I do silly things that no one understands. It doesn't really bother me, that they think I am weird. I am just in my own world, doing my own thing.

I had a lot of friends at my old school, I got to use my imagination a lot and it was easy grades kindergarten to first grade. I don't have any bad memories. Each year I was doing better at school. I didn't even know I had this Autistic thing. It wasn't until I was eight or nine years old my mom told me about it. I was getting depressed, sad, lonely, until one day I met the boy that would change my life. His name was Harper. We had so much fun. We played on his trampoline, in his treehouse, and at my house. We had so much fun together. It made my life a lot better and I was forgetting about the Autism. I learned I could

I LEARNED I COULD HAVE FUN AND MAKE FRIENDS.

have fun and make friends. I even ran for my school class president. I wanted to teach everyone about kids with disabilities. I was very successful and only lost by two votes!

JUST BE YOURSELF!

It is OK to have Autism, it is OK to remember it, but maybe you can just let it go and not even know that you have Autism. Just be yourself.

SIX

WHAT'S THE DEAL WITH THE GUT?

We have had so many challenges with Caden and his eating. When "gluten free" became the popular thing to do, so many people advised me I had to eliminate gluten from Caden's diet.

Like a lot of things, this sounded right, something I should do, could do, but it also made me anxious just thinking about it. I would have to clear out my entire kitchen, educate myself on what to look for on the backs of food packages, and, at the top of the to-do list, *cook*!

So, here's the reality: I don't cook. I like to bake sometimes, and I have a few go-to dishes I can cook pretty well—tacos, teriyaki chicken, avocado toast, and I make the best ceviche (after all, no cooking involved), and we can't forget the American favorite, hot dogs. But conjuring up some magnificent meals daily just makes me cringe.

Don't get me wrong—I did not just entertain the idea of cooking regularly, I actually tried several times, even attempting to organize meals for the week. All with little success. I just can't do it. I have zero patience for that chore. To the women who enjoy cooking, my hat goes off to you. Kudos! I think that is a talent.

That said, being the amazing cook that I am NOT, do you think I was ready to go gluten-free? Hell, no! So, for now, the cookbooks, which I continue to buy, continue to be decor for my kitchen.

When Caden was born, as with all parents, Tome and I were exhausted and in love with the new life we brought into this world. I had a C-section with all three of my boys, and my stay at the hospital was almost five days each time. Caden stayed in the room with me the entire time, except when nurses took him for normal tests in the nursery. One morning, a nurse asked when Caden had last had a bowel movement. I honestly couldn't remember. The nurse took Caden and, when she returned, proudly suggested that I should thank her. It turned out that she had to manually remove a blockage to allow his poop to come out. And it sure did work! I was thankful, very thankful, that I wasn't there to witness it.

The first few years of Caden's life were spent with a bottle in his mouth. He ate organic baby food and didn't seem to mind or dislike any variety of things I fed him. I remember he particularly liked sweet potatoes. We were given very strict orders from our pediatrician—once Caden turned two, we were to give him no more bottles. However, Caden loved his bottle, I mean *loved*! It was his comfort item. We used the old school Playtex bottles. He would suck all the air out of the bag in the bottle and toddle around the house, empty bottle—his "baba"—hanging from his mouth. For him, it was not just for the love of milk, it was soothing to him, his go-to security, much like a blanket or pacifier.

The minute his therapist knocked on the door for his morning session, the baba was in his mouth. Caden was up to four bottles a day. We waited another year when he was three to wean him. By then, we thought he would start drinking milk out of a sippy cup and decided to wean him cold turkey. We thought, surely he was old enough. Instead, as far as drinking milk went, we learned it was a bottle or nothing for him. Since that time, he has not had a single drop of milk. Talk about strong willed, or is this hard-headed? (Not sure where he gets that from—me?)

Caden started eating finger foods and was soon into breads and refried beans. He loved beans! We tried to feed him fruits and veggies, but he wasn't too interested and we didn't push. One afternoon, my husband was at work and I was home with Caden. He began whining and crying, and Caden rarely cried. I could tell he was trying to poop, but he couldn't.

Not only was he crying, he was *screaming*. He only did this when he was really in pain.

Up to this point, Caden had not had any stomach, digestion, constipation, or bowel issues. I had mostly forgotten about his episode in the hospital shortly after he was born. Now I had this screaming two-year-old, his face turning bright red, trying to poop, and screaming through tears and pain.

The first thing doctors will say in situations like this is to try prune juice or prunes. Obviously, they don't know my child, because that wasn't happening.

I called my husband in panic. I filled the tub with warm water and put him in the bath. They say warm water can move your bowels. Screaming, screaming, and more screaming, almost as if the water was burning him. I am going to be brief and as non-descriptive as possible, but I basically had to help him get this blocked poop out. What came out was a golf ball! Not literally, of course, but it was the size of a golf ball and almost as hard. I could not believe that for the past couple hours, poor Caden was trying to get this out of his little body. And I could not believe I had to stick my finger up my baby's ass and get a poo ball out. Such fond memories.

This was the beginning of our realization and awareness that Caden had issues with food and his gut.

CADEN HAD ISSUES WITH FOOD AND HIS GUT!

As Caden grew, I realized the critical importance of nutrients he needed to be a healthy kid. As parents, we are supposed to provide balanced meals for our children, taking from all the food groups: fruits and vegetables, proteins, carbs and so on. We were taught this when we were children ourselves, and even though things have shifted a little, the basics are still true.

Unfortunately, Caden despised fruits and vegetables, every single one. He hated that I even put them on his plate. I would go through cycles, trying different ways to introduce various "new" fruits to him, but he wanted nothing to do with it. At first, I didn't push him. His pediatrician seemed to think that was OK, and that his taste buds would change as he got older. In other words, as he grew up, Caden would be more open to eating fruits and vegetables. Or so the doctor said. I'm still waiting for this momentous occasion.

In the middle of setting goals for therapy, Caden's eating habits were brought up, including introducing fruits and vegetables. I was doubtful, but I figured we could at least try. Caden's therapist would show up for

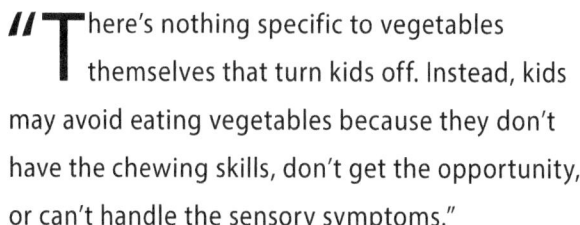

// There's nothing specific to vegetables themselves that turn kids off. Instead, kids may avoid eating vegetables because they don't have the chewing skills, don't get the opportunity, or can't handle the sensory symptoms."

—Jenny Friedman, Autism nutritionist

a session with an assortment of fruits (we started with fruits as they are sweeter and perhaps an easier challenge to tackle). Caden entertained us as she cut up the fruit and placed pieces on a plate. She sat with Caden at the table, but after days of watching a frustrated toddler waste hours of therapy and accomplishing nothing, I made the decision to pull this "goal" from his program for the time being. There were so many other important things to work on instead, like daily functioning skills, so I decided to pick my battles and move forward.

> "YOU'RE AMAZING, BUT YOU CAN'T DO IT ALL."

Our days of therapy continued, and my thoughts of becoming a chef wouldn't leave my mind. Any day now this cooking would kick in, I would kid myself. It was comical. One week I would be so busy that everything we ate came from our favorite Mexican restaurant, the one and only El Gringo, and the next week I was spending $30 for a piece of wild halibut and trying to come up with a fancy way to cook broccoli so my kids would like it. I was all over the place, and Caden was still an all-bean eater.

Don't get me wrong, beans are good for you, but they can't be the only thing you eat. As I continued talking to other moms, therapists, professionals, and teachers, I was gaining so much knowledge. I learned how the gut is like a second brain and affects many of our functions. That was eye opening and so interesting, it made so much sense to me.

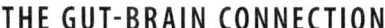

THE GUT-BRAIN CONNECTION

The gut is sometimes referred to as our second brain! The physical connection of the Gut and the Brain is via the Vagus nerve. This is a neural superhighway second only to the spinal column. Embedded in the wall of the gut, is the enteric nervous system (ENS) that controls digestion to some degree. Neurons in the gut are thought to generate as much Dopamine as those in the head, and 90% of our Serotonin is produced in the gut. Mood is inextricably linked to gut health. We are all familiar with the idea of feeling sick to the stomach with worry or anxiety, as well as feeling butterflies in the stomach over a new date!

—Good 4 the Gut

The link between digestive problems and Autism is undeniable, and it's related to inflammatory bowel issues, acid reflux within the gastrointestinal tract, and possibly more. This is partially due to the inflammation that food allergies and digestive issues can bring on, which can be painful and influence behavior negatively.

This brain-gut link also puts these children at risk of nutritional deficiencies, which can aggravate cognition problems and adversely affect immune responses.

"Early life environmental factors can also play a part in the development of Autism Spectrum Disorder. The study cites prenatal and postnatal diet, gut microbiota, and immune system triggers as contributors to the disorder's prevalence."

—Julie Matthews, *Nourishing Hope*

I knew what I needed to do—start a new life routine with my family—and I knew it had to start with me. This time, I was all in.

Change is scary; it is the unknown. It can be overwhelming and cause major anxiety. I was feeling all of it. I am so thankful that just when I needed it, I was introduced to a local mother/daughter team, the Curry Girls, who just happened to be neighbors of my childhood best friend.

The Curry Girls, self-described healthy-food crusaders, helped clean me out, literally and in my kitchen. After meeting with them to discuss my health concerns for myself and my family, we started to eliminate various foods from my family's diet. We scoured my pantry and cabinets, eliminating not only toxic foods, but Teflon pans and any cooking utensils that could release chemicals into our food.

It was at this time I decided I was ready to try this gluten-free eating phenomenon. I needed to eliminate gluten to see what effects it would have on all of us. I kept hearing that kids were being "cured" of Autism because gluten was eliminated from their diets. It made sense to me that certain foods might be harmful or toxic, and that people could naturally be predisposed to be intolerant to them or even allergic. Take that out of anyone's diet, one is bound to see positive results.

I wasn't going to take on every change that needed to happen in my life at one time. Baby steps were needed, maybe even crawling.

Remember: I am not a cook, so of course I was freaking out about going gluten-free. What was I going to cook? What would my kids eat? Gluten is in so many ingredients, and you really have to know how to read and interpret labels. To my relief, the Curry Girls started to deliver home-cooked dinners three times a week. At least I was guaranteed to feed my family three meals that were not only gluten-free but filled with the nutrients they needed.

That was the spearhead of my exploration to discover what the deal was with the gut. As I mentioned above, I'd been told the stomach is our second brain and everything that we eat affects us. Clean the gut, clear the brain.

CLEAN THE GUT, CLEAR THE BRAIN.

I was starting to get it. I wasn't going to be a totally obsessed psycho-mom who wouldn't allow my kids to live—they are kids, for heaven's sake—but the food in my house would be clean. I could control what they ate at home and allow them to eat what they wanted when they were at a friend's house or a birthday party.

Soon they learned their own bodies and how different foods made them feel, including horrible stomach pain and headaches from sugar. One night, we went to my kids' favorite restaurant for one of their birthday dinners. By that time, my boys had been eating clean and sugar-free for a few weeks. I allowed them each a glass of lemonade, but Caden snuck in a few more free refills. To be honest, I didn't care too much, they had been so good with all "Mom's new rules." Like a light switch, Caden went from coloring with his crayons on the menu to coloring on his face! Like someone who just got an overdose of adrenaline, he was out of control. What the hell was going on? It did not take long to realize that the sugar was hitting his bloodstream, and all we could do was sit wide-eyed, looking at each other.

Over the next few years, we could see the effects food had on our kids. It was clear that everything we consume affects our mood, energy, focus, ability to sit still, and what it does to our inside

> **IT WAS CLEAR THAT EVERYTHING WE CONSUME AFFECTS OUR MOOD, ENERGY, FOCUS, ABILITY TO SIT STILL.**

is a whole other story. I am a believer! I have seen the effects of what we put in our bodies, into our gut. Did you know, 70 percent of our serotonin—which directly affects our mood, anxiety, depression, and focus—is produced in our gut? Pretty amazing.

In general, we put our lives and our well-being in the hands of doctors, relying heavily on their diagnoses and advice. Doctors are trained to look for symptoms and signs of anything that may be affecting a patient, then they make their diagnoses and advise and prescribe. They are doing what they know. But never once has a doctor brought to my attention that the food my kids are consuming may significantly change their behavior and ability to function (besides eating the normal fruits and vegetables, getting enough calcium etc.). This is where I feel our society has failed. There are some amazing doctors; I am not saying they are bad. What I am suggesting is that we need to be more diligent to educate ourselves in order to make the best decisions for our children.

I mentioned earlier that Caden has a high pain tolerance. When he is crying from pain, I know it is bad. One weekend, Tome called me in a panic. Caden was lying on the couch, curled up and screaming. I, of course, did what I normally do and freaked out, knowing Caden never complained of pain. I rushed home and found Caden exactly as Tome had said. The way he was screaming and crying and asking me to make it stop, I thought it was his appendix. But that was ruled out when I realized the pain was on the wrong side.

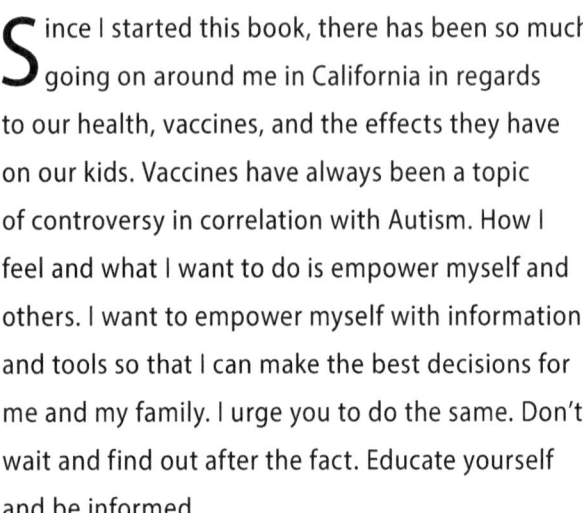

Since I started this book, there has been so much going on around me in California in regards to our health, vaccines, and the effects they have on our kids. Vaccines have always been a topic of controversy in correlation with Autism. How I feel and what I want to do is empower myself and others. I want to empower myself with information and tools so that I can make the best decisions for me and my family. I urge you to do the same. Don't wait and find out after the fact. Educate yourself and be informed.

We knew right away we had to get him to an emergency room. Cut to the point, Caden's severe abdominal pain was the result of gas and constipation, which the doctor said could be excruciating. That was the last episode we have had—one more impetus to be even more diligent and aware of what we eat.

So, where are we today? Caden still does not eat fruits and vegetables. Don't judge. I do what I can. This kid can find the tiniest bit of any fruit or veggie, no matter how I try to hide it. When I can get him to take a few bites here and there, I always loudly praise him. We discovered "That's It" fruit and veggie bars that contain two different things per bar. That's it! He will usually eat one if I basically tell him he is going to die from lack of nutrients. It's ironic that this kid, who watches every how-to video on YouTube and follows what they say, still has a hard time with food. He loves science and was really into Magic School Bus videos for a while. After every video, he would sit and tell me all about the insides of our bodies and how the kidney functions and why we need it. He also watched the episode on nutrition, but somehow it just didn't stick. Go figure.

I continue to pick my battles with Caden and food, making sure we are aware of all the foods he is eating; nothing (for the most part) processed, no refined sugars, and lots of water. This, along with vitamins and supplements, has gotten us through until now. I have to take it day by day and hope that he will come around to understand the importance of good nutrition. Mind over matter, right? He definitely has something in his mind that all fruits and veggies are bad.

"Caden, seriously, what is it with the fruits and veggies? Is it the taste? Is it the texture? What is it?"

His answer, as always, was unexpected: "Mom, I just think it is weird you can turn them into juice." I am still digesting this one.

SEVEN

FINDING THE LIGHT

No one wants to be labeled. No one. And we especially don't want that for our children. **NO ONE WANTS TO BE LABELED.** No two people are exactly alike in this world, so why categorize and generalize who we are as people? We are supposed to be individuals and stand out. Unfortunately, our world is very judgmental, and being different is not always accepted.

    The day we received two-year-old Caden's diagnosis was the day our lives changed. Forever. Although we did not know what we were doing, or if the path we were taking was the right one, we hit the ground running full speed ahead and never looked back.

    There were so many therapies and resources to discover and so much research to be done, it was difficult to navigate, and there was no crystal ball to peer into. I held my son's future successes in my hands but I had no idea what I was doing and there was no one to guide me—it all felt overwhelming and filled me with increasing anxiety. But I didn't have a choice. I knew Caden had amazing things in store, and I was bound and determined to help him find his path.

Yes, there are experts and doctors who can advise you. But it's *your* job to help your child. You *must* be an advocate for him in a world that doesn't make it easy. It's a scary responsibility.

Everyone has an opinion, even those who have no right to say anything about Autism. There are about 4 million results if you google "high functioning Autism." It's up to *you* to weed through all the "noise" and figure out what will help your child.

We received some direction from the Regional Center. Brace yourself as I introduce you to a lot of acronyms. They had us contact PTN (Pediatric Therapy Network), which provides ST (speech therapy), OT (occupational therapy), PT (physical therapy), and consultation. PTN's mission is to lead the way in helping children, families, and communities reach full capabilities through innovative therapy, education, and research programs.

I held Caden's chubby two-year-old hand as we walked through the PTN doors for the first time. I will never forget this experience. The woman at the front desk told me that his class was all the way at the end of the building and to walk through the doors until I got there. Door after door, we entered a new class, and then exited. Every nerve in my body was on edge.

The children we encountered as we popped in and out of classrooms were severe cases. There was so much commotion and chaos everywhere with kids yelling and crying. The sounds were *loud*! My anxiety climbed to an all-time high, and I felt my throat closing up till I could barely breathe. I am sure my senses were heightened. Some kids sat quietly, others rocked back and forth as they moaned. Caden wanted to stare as a little boy was kicking and screaming because he didn't want to wash his hands. Caden feels things deeper than most. He does not like to see others in pain, ever, emotionally or physically.

> **WHEN YOU JUDGE SOMEONE BASED ON THEIR DIAGNOSIS, YOU MISS OUT ON THEIR ABILITIES, BEAUTY AND UNIQUENESS.**

I couldn't stop feeling scared as we walked through each room. I didn't even realize when I picked my baby up and held him close in my arms, as if I needed to protect him. My initial thought was that he didn't belong here.

I've heard that when you witness others worse off than you, you feel a certain amount of gratefulness. Well, I didn't get that feeling at all. I was saddened deeply to see so many children physically unable to

> "As we all want our children, both boys and girls, to have every opportunity to flourish into the person they are meant to become, it's vital that we stop labeling and acknowledge room for growth, change and reinvention."
> —Dr. Robyn Silverman

share their gifts. Would they ever be able to? Was this therapy the answer?

Feeling helpless and hopeful at the same time can be a scary place. We finally reached the last door, and when we entered I was taken aback. There were five other boys, around the same age as Caden all sitting at a little table doing puzzles. It was quiet, calm, and peaceful. These boys were all content. My nerves began to lessen and I put Caden down to join them. They allowed me to stay for Caden's first class, watching him smile as they finger painted and jumped into a ball pit. I still wasn't sure if this was where he actually fit, but at least it was a start.

THE THERAPY ROAD TRAVELED

ABA (Applied Behavior Analysis) is "a scientific discipline concerned with applying techniques based upon the principles of learning to change behavior of social significance." From the time of diagnosis until Caden was eight years old, we had therapists in our house most of every day. In his first year, before he turned three, his schedule was tiresome. The first therapist would knock on the door at 8:30 a.m. sharp. Caden would run to his room and grab his blankie and bottle for comfort. The "shift" lasted four hours. Caden would then get a small nap break, or maybe a trip to the park

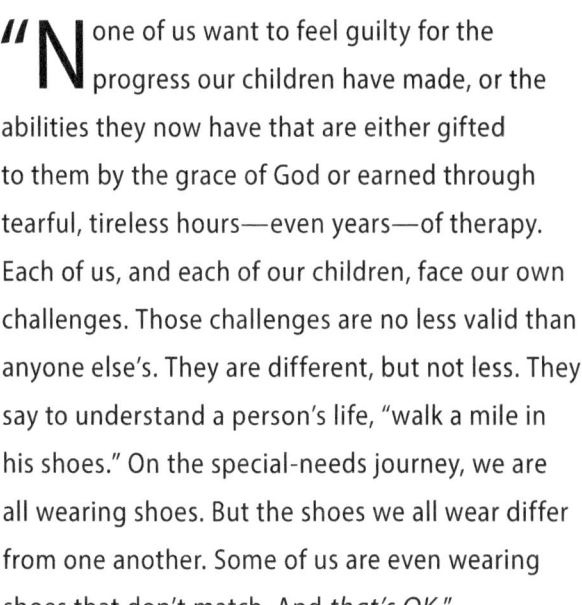

"None of us want to feel guilty for the progress our children have made, or the abilities they now have that are either gifted to them by the grace of God or earned through tearful, tireless hours—even years—of therapy. Each of us, and each of our children, face our own challenges. Those challenges are no less valid than anyone else's. They are different, but not less. They say to understand a person's life, "walk a mile in his shoes." On the special-needs journey, we are all wearing shoes. But the shoes we all wear differ from one another. Some of us are even wearing shoes that don't match. And *that's OK*."

—Sarah, Specialneedsparenting.net

or the grocery store. Then therapist number two would arrive and stay from 2:30 until 6:30 p.m.

I always felt terrible for whoever had the second shift. Caden was exhausted by then. He had worked hard all morning, and he let it be known in toddler fashion how done he was when the second person arrived. Truth is, I think I had a harder time with all of this structured and intrusive learning than Caden did. The constant parade of therapists, day in and day out, meant there was zero privacy for me. Therapists heard every phone conversation, knew what I was doing at all times, and saw me too many times in my PJs or just coming out of the shower.

I used to call ABA therapy a "parroting" session. *Caden, say this, Caden, do this. Nope, do it again, but this time looking at me. Can you hold this pencil, Caden? Can you draw a straight line, Caden?* This was all day, every day. It was exhausting just listening; how could my son not feel the same?

"You won't be perfect, that's a guarantee. But it's hard to not *try* to make it perfect when it's your child at stake. And then to not feel guilty when something fails."

—Livingwellmom.com

I have never been much of a reader or a researcher. I am a talker. I get all my information from people and their experiences. I like to see and read people's emotions when I am in conversations, it can be so telling. Every therapy I have ever had my kids in is because I have learned what it did for another kid and I had to try it. I learn from others' stories and experiences.

When you have a kid with special needs, or any type of need, Google does not always have your best interest at heart—it's impersonal. I started Caden at both Neuro-Fit and Neuro-Zone because of recommendations from other moms. These two forms of therapy did amazing things for not only Caden, but for Kyle as well.

> **RELAX, WE'RE ALL CRAZY. IT'S NOT A COMPETITION.**

Neuro-Fit was awesome. This was a physical therapy, one of the very few therapies Caden looked forward to. Neuro-Fit states, "We help people who struggle, improve their coordination and brain's processing speeds, by reducing nerve system stress and overload in our twelve-week, medication-free, movement protocol." What did this actually mean? I had no clue. However, I began to understand the process a little.

We have a symmetrical midline that runs vertically down our bodies, including our brains. The exercises they had Caden doing crossed from one side of the body to the other, causing neurons to fire. Once they could get them to fire, they would start to connect one to another, and the body would have those connections permanently.

This facility was more or less a gym with a roll-up garage door. Caden would climb on top of a huge tractor tire, balancing as his therapist threw dodge balls at him, one to the left, then one to the right. He did a lot of exercises hopping on one foot, reaching his right hand to the opposite foot, and one of his favorites was being shot across the turf on a sled by what looked like a large slingshot.

Caden's balance and coordination definitely improved. Like everything else, this was a huge expense for us, and we could only afford it for a year. The distance was also an issue as it was not close to our house. This was typical of all the therapies—expensive and usually inconvenient. We would give them a certain amount of time, see improvement, and then move onto something new. To this day, Caden still asks to go back to Neuro-Fit.

Speech therapy, occupational therapy, cognitive behavior therapy, educational therapy, social interaction adaptive therapy, the list goes on and on. Caden loves OT, most of the time. This is all motor skills and sensory regulation exercises. He gets to make obstacle courses and play in the ball pit, which he loves. He does not love practicing holding his pencil correctly or printing.

It wasn't until last year that I started having Caden do OT outside of school on a more intense level. I knew that he had always had sensory issues, I just didn't realize to what extent. There are two types of sensory processing. One

"I DON'T NEED EASY, I JUST NEED POSSIBLE."

—BETHANY HAMILTON

is when the body receives too much input and can't process it at all. These are kids who, for example, can't tolerate tags in their clothes, usually don't like to touch slime or odd textures, aren't fans of foods that are sticky or too smooth or perhaps even the smell. Sounds are also overwhelming, lights can be too bright; they are basically on sensory overload.

Our brains depend on precise processing of sensory information to create maps of our body, our environment, and how we fit into the world. If you want to pick up a glass of water, you need to know where your hand is on your body, where your hand is relative to the glass, and where the glass is on the table. Accurate processing of information is also vital to how we interact in our world socially and behaviorally. When our brain isn't breaking down the stimulation properly, our senses can't interpret the information correctly.
        —Innova Brain Rehabilitation

Some kids seem to have trouble handling the information their senses take in—things like sound, touch, taste, sight, and smell. Besides these common senses, there are also two other less well-known ones that can be affected—*proprioception*, or a sense of body awareness, and *vestibular* sense, which involves movement, balance, and coordination.

Kids with sensory-processing issues experience too much or too little stimulation through these senses. They may also have difficulty integrating sensory information—for example things that they see and hear simultaneously, like a person speaking—might seem out of sync for them.

These problems can be tough on kids, and get in the way of them functioning effectively, learning, and making friends.

Sensory-processing problems tend to come in two types, under- and over-sensitivity, although it's common for one child to experience both kinds.

Hypersensitive kids are extremely reactive to sensory stimulation and can find it overwhelming. They may:

- Be unable to tolerate bright lights and loud noises like ambulance sirens
- Be distracted by background noises that others don't seem to hear
- Refuse to wear clothing because it feels scratchy or irritating—even after cutting out all the tags and labels—or shoes because they feel "too tight"

- Be fearful of surprise touch, avoid hugs and cuddling even with familiar adults
- Be overly fearful of swings and playground equipment
- Often have trouble understanding where their body is in relation to other objects or people
- Bump into things and appear clumsy
- Have trouble sensing the amount of force they're applying; for example, they may rip the paper when erasing, pinch too hard or slam objects down.

Hyposensitive kids are under-sensitive, which makes them want to seek out *more* sensory stimulation. They may:

- Have a constant need to touch people or textures, even when it's not socially acceptable
- Not understand personal space even when kids the same age are old enough to understand it
- Have an extremely high tolerance for pain
- Not understand their own strength
- Be very fidgety and unable to sit still
- Love jumping, bumping and crashing activities
- Enjoy deep pressure like tight bear hugs
- Crave fast, spinning, and/or intense movement
- Love being tossed in the air and jumping on furniture and trampolines.

—Child Mind Institute

Then there is the other kind of sensory processing, the kind Caden has. He is a kid who needs more input. I like to explain it this way to people: If you or I were to put a hand on a hot stove, we yanked it away quickly, feeling the heat or burning sensation within seconds. This is automatic. If Caden were to touch the stove, he would have to use his cognitive skills, telling himself that the stove is hot and he probably should pull his hand away. His body does not receive enough input to tell his muscles to respond and act. This is an extreme example, and untrue for Caden. However, this is very true for many other situations for him.

In 2018, when Caden was in the fifth grade, he learned to hold onto a monkey bar and "wheelbarrow" across the room. Swimming has been a challenge—floppy arms and his motoring legs are weak. I am happy to report that his strokes are looking great, and he can swim a lap in 30 seconds. This is a huge accomplishment.

For Caden, even sitting up is difficult. Gravity pulls us down; our body feels that and tells our brain, which communicates to our muscles to sit up straight. Caden doesn't receive those messages. His brain to muscle transmission is very weak. When I learned that it took 80 percent of his focus and energy just to sit up at his desk, I was blown away. I actually had a moment, thinking how far he had come academically with only 20 percent of his ability to focus. Caden will sit, but he is like a soda can being shaken up. He can only do it so long, and then he bursts.

He will take occasional breaks throughout the day to walk around the school. He needs this, and kids don't understand why. I asked his therapist why he can sit at the computer for hours, and that doesn't seem difficult. She told me it was a preferred task for him, and when he has his tablet, phone, and computer on at the same time, they all function at the pace of his brain, so he is able to focus and maintain. But he does get up after a while and goes right to the trampoline to jump.

Caden falls into the hyposensitive category. All his behaviors through the years make sense now. I did have an "I'm a terrible parent" moment, thinking I should have had him in intensive OT years ago, but the truth is that Caden would not have been ready for it then. There is a process. You can't put the horse before the carriage. All that matters is that he is getting what he needs now. I can only worry about today.

TO MEDICATE OR NOT

There is an entire other side to helping our children, which includes medications, essential oils, CBD oil, tinctures, vitamins, and so on. We have tried them all.

I was never keen on medicating my kids. I understand the possible benefits and have no problem making that decision for myself as an adult, but when it comes to my children, medications become a scary thought. I struggled for a very long time always wondering about meds and the possibilities of helping

Caden. Every couple of years, I would bring it up to the boys' pediatrician.

She always said the same thing: "It is not a tattoo, it's not permanent. If you try them (medications) and they aren't working, you can stop using them." I sat with those words, the thought of "what if?" sitting on one shoulder. What if we used it, and we saw a huge change? What if? I had been living with "what if?" for years, and that feeling was not going away. When Caden was in the fourth grade, after I listened to friends' stories about how it helped their kids, I had to give meds a try.

Let's just say medication therapy lasted about a month.

On the first day, Caden sat down and read for 60 minutes straight. He put a timer on and read for the entire time. He had never done that before. His focus was definitely better, but he was not the same Caden. It was like we lost him. His personality was not the same, his humor was gone, all the things that made Caden who he was disappeared.

> **HIS PERSONALITY WAS NOT THE SAME, HIS HUMOR WAS GONE.**

He was snippy and would talk back, things he had never done before. Teachers were seeing the same things at school. It was amazing to me, though, how conspicuous the change was. We didn't tell his teachers of our planned experimental approach, and the very same day we started him on meds, that exact day, I got a call from one of his teachers asking if we had put him on meds. I mean, that is crazy, right?

The personality change was obvious. So I checked meds off the box. I know meds work for some, and there are those who really do need them. I am not against the use of drug therapy, it just isn't right for Caden.

Searching for alternative medicines can be difficult, and the trust level in your doctor is important. Stories were haunting me about doctors coming up with "cures" for Autism or even cancer, and then mysteriously being found dead in a river after committing suicide. I could not believe how powerful our pharmaceutical companies were, and that money—the root of all evil—does really control the world.

By this time, I had found a natural doctor who was doing "underground medicine." I didn't even know what that meant, I just knew it was something I shouldn't talk about. I am a believer in how things are meant to happen. My journey has taken me to some amazing places and has allowed me to meet people who have changed my life. I am always open, allowing opportunity to come my way.

My encounter with this doctor was no accident, it was meant to be. Because I am very open about my life, my kids, and who I am, I allow people in. They feel safe with me. When I shared with this doctor about my family, she knew she had to help me, and she did. She described her medicines and how they could help not only Caden but our entire family.

We were all tested and were so surprised by the results. Parasites, vitamin deficiency, candida, viruses of all kinds—we had no clue what was going on inside our bodies. We decided to do a vitamin and metal test to see what deficiencies we had and what metals were in our bodies. This included allergy testing as well. It is mind-blowing what you can learn.

Anyway, we started taking tinctures. The bottles came in, and we each had a bag. The colors varied from green to yellow and brown. The labels on each bottle were fictitious. Because this medicine was underground, everything had to be made up. We took home our tinctures and every morning and night we would put the prescribed number of drops into our drinks. We did this for more than a year, without missing a dose. I was nuts about it. Teachers, even the principal, came up to me and asked what I was doing with Caden—they had noticed such a difference with him. I think it was a combination of the tinctures, therapies, and diet we had been putting him on. When we were re-tested and our numbers where we wanted them to be, we stopped with the tinctures but continued eating clean, knowing how we are affected by what we put into our bodies.

> TEACHERS, EVEN THE PRINCIPAL, NOTICED A DIFFERENCE WITH CADEN.

Therapies can be endless, and there are so many great resources out there, but not many are talked about and shared. I have a hard time with the expense of it all. I would do anything for my kids, especially to help them succeed and live happy, healthy lives. It seems like a lot of the things in this world are only easily accessible to the wealthy. If you want to live a clean, non-GMO, organic, healthy lifestyle, your bills will go up.

Kids with special needs struggle every day in many ways. They have to work harder than most, and spend their time in therapy instead of playing with friends. They have a hard time in school, with motor functions, sensory issues, and social situations.

As a parent, I do the best I can to make it easier, to give light to a path that will allow Caden to spread his wings and fly. I know there are amazing places he can go and opportunities around the corner, but they all come at an enormous expense. So, on top of all the obstacles that come with Autism, there is nothing more stressful and heartbreaking than knowing that I can't always afford to help my child. Why is that? Why do the government and insurance companies make everything so difficult? I doubt that I will ever have an answer to that question.

> I DO THE BEST I CAN TO LIGHT A PATH THAT WILL ALLOW CADEN TO SPREAD HIS WINGS AND FLY.

My stress level is high, and my emotions are raw. The one thing that is in my power is to put positive energy out into the world every day, hopeful that good things will come our way, prayerful that we will catch a break, that the little glimmer at the end of the tunnel will grow brighter as we continue this journey together.

I will never give up.

EIGHT

QUEEN OF THE CASTLE

For as long as I can remember, I have always been a helper. I run to the aid of anyone who has a problem that needs solving, or who needs an ear to listen or a shoulder to cry on. I would go out of my way to make someone feel better when sad or going through a tough time. As I got older, I gradually realized that this behavior was filling a void.

As women and mothers, by nature, we put ourselves last. We take care of our husbands and children, and if there is a free hour to spare, we may meet a girlfriend for a glass of wine or take a much needed nap. We will fit in an occasional massage, haircut, facial, or buy ourselves a new pair of jeans, but these are all temporary "highs." So, we look good, play the part, make ourselves believe we are all OK. Or maybe it's someone like me: I move too fast to allow my brain to realize I'm actually not all OK.

Am I being selfish? I thought about this as I lay in bed one night, a million "to dos" going through my head as usual. I was tired of feeling like a hamster on a wheel, of not feeling like I had a purpose. I was tired of giving excuses. I needed passion. I needed a reason to get up every morning, beyond making lunches and beds or kissing my husband goodbye as he left for work. What the hell was I doing with my life?

It was time for me to get to know myself again and discover who I was and what I wanted in my life. How could I encourage my sons to make this journey if I was not willing?

> SOMETIMES YOU DON'T REALIZE YOU'RE ACTUALLY DROWNING WHEN YOU ARE TRYING TO BE EVERYONE ELSE'S ANCHOR.

I began soul searching, which scared the crap out of me. I knew this meant I had to spend time with myself, get to know myself, and I wasn't sure I was ready.

I was so lost, I really didn't know what to do. I needed direction and guidance, so I called my friends to do an energy reading on me. I learned a lot that day. I learned that I am intuitive and can foresee things. Of course, learning this, I immediately started second-guessing everything I was doing. I came to the realization that I could only control today. Tomorrow was something new, and I needed to trust and believe that my path was there. I just needed to open my eyes and heart to accept what was being given to me.

I began writing down all my thoughts and feelings that I had held inside for years. It was therapeutic and emotional. I was reliving pieces of my life, really feeling for the first time. I would read stories I wrote to my husband and I would get choked up as feelings overwhelmed me. This was something new for me, something I had never allowed to enter my soul. As I wrote one story after the next, my eyes were opening, and I was slowly seeing the person I was and the person I am and will be.

> **I JUST NEEDED TO OPEN MY EYES AND HEART TO ACCEPT WHAT WAS BEING GIVEN TO ME.**

As I helped others, moms of kids with special needs or struggles, I was simultaneously helping myself. I created a safe place for us to share and be vulnerable without being judged.

We are connected, and that understanding and compassion run deep. There is an unspoken bond between us, and it is strong.

I sought something deeper, more meaningful, in my life. With my eyes open, I was seeing the world in a new light. Opportunities and people were coming to me, and I wondered if they had been there all along, unseen. One day, I was drawn to something a friend discussed on Facebook. I really didn't know what she was talking about, but it was inspiring and I wanted more. After contacting her and learning what she was doing, I signed up to get my life-coaching certificate.

The work I did over the next year was life changing. I learned more about myself than I ever thought possible. I learned about boundaries and values and about believing in and loving myself. I set goals and had a vision for my future, a life's mission statement that is powerful. I recognized who added to my life and who brought negative energy, who was worthy of being allowed into my world and who I didn't need to share with. I learned the difference between love and compassion, empathy and sympathy, and I am no longer afraid to feel. The feelings I had pushed down for so long were all surfacing, and they weren't scary to face after all.

I was ready. I was strong and courageous and ready to face my fears.

I WAS READY... STRONG AND COURAGEOUS AND READY TO FACE MY FEARS.

I slowly pulled away from a career that had been looming over me for years. I needed the money it provided so I could pay for therapy and doctor bills, but it was slowly eating away at me. I wasn't being who I was on the inside. I needed to find my passion, my purpose. I felt an energy pulling me, leading me to do something more.

I knew change for my family needed to start with me. Taking a huge leap of faith and following my heart,

I jumped. I jumped in by taking care of my body, inside and out. We have always been a pretty clean family, eating organic and limiting sugar and dairy. What I put into my body wasn't my problem—it was my daily consumption and habits. I was not raised with the best role model for an eater. I am a snacker—little snacks throughout the day, no big meals.

I was tired of worrying about everything I put in my mouth. Food still controlled me the way it always had. I eat more now than I ever have, yet, in my forties, I am healthier than I have ever been. I have given myself time each day to workout, because I want to and it makes me feel good. I need it to relieve stress, to make my body feel good, and to know that I am doing something good for my health.

I am still trying to balance the triangle of kids, husband, and me time. Nourishing my relationship is something I have worked to put more time into. Tome, my husband, my partner, is my person. I have learned that if I open up and share everything that I used to hold in and carry alone, it not only makes me lighter, but brings us closer together. We are a team.

I continue to battle with the friendships and people in my life, recognizing those I choose to spend time with and which relationships I want to invest in. There are days when I feel I have no friends, days when I feel I have too many, and days when I want none at all. I teeter back and forth with invites for book clubs and moms' night out, old friends, new friends, working relationships, and people I actually *want* to get to know. There is just not enough time, and I have learned when to say no.

Stepping outside my comfort zone has been the hardest thing for me. I think it is the hardest thing for most people. I have put myself out there. I am being vulnerable, being my true self. It is freeing and empowering to be who I am 100 percent and to be proud of every ounce of my being, imperfections and all.

I am looking within and discovering strength I never knew I had before. I am learning I have a voice—I have something to say, and I want to share with others. I don't want to be overshadowed or stepped on or overlooked or walked over. I want to be seen and heard and loved and appreciated. I want to teach my boys to be authentic and proud and never pretend to be anything but who they are.

Start each day with a smile on your face and a song in your heart. That is what my mom used to tell me. If you wake up making the choice to have a good day, it is impossible to start off on the wrong foot. I am trying to slow down and enjoy the small moments. I am used to running full speed, I feel like my life is always in fast forward. My brain is constantly spinning, and I am consciously trying to make that stop, to be present and breathe.

I meditated for the first time recently. Those who know me know that sitting still is an accomplishment all on its own. I tell people, "If you see me sitting on the couch watching TV, I'm dying." Meditation is something I have wanted to do, but I knew it would be very uncomfortable and challenging. It was worth the wait, because I had the most amazing experience. I am motivated to carve out ten minutes each day to be quiet and still.

The life I have been given is not easy. No one has it easy. I have three boys who are all unique in their own ways and come with challenges. They have filled my life with color and my heart with more emotion and feeling than I thought possible. My

> **THEY FILL MY LIFE WITH COLOR AND MY HEART WITH MORE EMOTION AND FEELING THAN I THOUGHT POSSIBLE.**

husband loves me, sometimes more than I feel I deserve. He tries to give me everything I want to make me happy, even if it may not be in our best interest financially. What he doesn't realize is that he has already given me everything I want.

Having kids with special needs and having financial difficulties are two major causes for divorce. Tome and I are solid. We have our occasional ups and downs like everyone, which only make us stronger. Going through hard times, being able to support one another, to truly be a rock for the other, makes every hard time doable together.

So, as I continue to work on discovering me, allowing time to be selfish, I am healing. I am becoming a better mom to my boys, a better partner to my husband, and a better person to all.

I am becoming the best version of me.

NINE

LITTLE BOY WONDER

Maguire. Where do I start with telling you about this kid? Maguire was meant to be the third brother in this family. God knows just how to fit all the pieces of the family puzzle together.

Maguire was a baby born into therapy. He spent the first two years of his life listening to therapists teach Caden. We would joke that he was going to be so smart because he was seriously paying attention. Little did we know the power of our words.

MAGUIRE WAS BORN INTO THERAPY

Maguire also came into this world with more charisma than I know what to do with at times. He is wise beyond his years and always wants to do things on his own. He held his own bottle at three months old, ran before he walked, would hang from the monkey bars, and climb structures way too early.

Some may consider him a daredevil, however, I know for a fact he just has an uncanny knack to mimic everything with a dose of fearlessness. Since I can remember, Maguire would watch and listen intently to everything that was going on around him.

At parks, while kids would run and play, Maguire would sit and watch the older boys, soaking it all in just like a sponge. The next day, he would be doing exactly what those older boys had done, to a tee, move for move. Maguire still does not miss a beat! Nothing, and I mean nothing, gets by this kid.

He is off the wall an extrovert, breaking out in song and dance, being a total goofball. I often say, "I don't know where he gets that from." Then my best friend, Lindsay (who knows me better than all), says, "YOU! He gets it from you; he is *exactly* like you!"

Guess there's no denying, it's true, I am a total nerd, dork, goofball, and that cemented why Maguire and I have a special bond. We can sit for hours in my bed and belly laugh like you do with a school friend. The kind of laughing where you stop for a second, look at each other, and then uncontrollably laugh some more. We have a deep understanding for one another. He loves his mom, and when I say loves, if he could crawl back inside me, I think he would.

Maguire, of course, will always be my "baby," my last born, and that birth position holds its own special place in my heart, just as the others do in their birth order. However, I also recognize the inherent drawbacks of being my mini-me as he is also a little possessive when it comes to his mom. Seriously, Maguire will call me over and over and over again if I am out having some adult time. This has gotten a lot better, as he's getting older.

He would leave me messages that I would sometimes play for whomever I was with. "Come on, Mom, you have to pick up. Why do you have to go out with your friends anyway? This is the second time this week. Mom, you promised you would be home early, it's already nine… come on, Mom…" This coming from a, then, five-year-old. You get my drift? This just cannot be normal.

I would come home from the evening to find him curled up by the front door fast asleep in his blanket. I mean, how could I get mad? His care for me melts my heart. However, I am trying to find the balance between devoting every second I have to my kids before they are all grown up, to spending a little quality time with my husband, and not feeling guilty for carving out some free me time. The struggle is real!

When Maguire was in preschool, if there was an argument or scuffle between his classmates (boys, of course), the teacher would always call on my tiny "adult" to tell her what happened. Not only could he articulate every word, he could retell the situation like rewinding a video. His memory and what he retains are truly amazing! Every adult conversation, anything on TV, all absorbed. This sometimes is a bad thing, too, as he eavesdrops on my phone conversations or adult interactions, and if it's bad he is digesting that, too!

He is the person who walks into a room and it lights up. Maguire is "that" kid. He is nice to everyone and remembers children's names that he has only met once, never passing someone without a hello as he walks by. I can remember a time when his older brothers were at the elementary school and Maguire was still in preschool, we would walk the halls and the older kids were all drawn to him. I often overheard "There's Maguire!" "Cool socks, Maguire!" "That kid is so cool!" Really?!

Teachers love him as well. He does well in school and is such a perfectionist. If you have a child who is a perfectionist, you know this is *not* fun. I can't tell you how many pictures or cards we have drawn and with one little mistake, in the trash it goes. Hours and hours spent on getting it just right. Yikes!

Parents, too, are taken with Maguire. I've been told on more than one occasion that he is going to be president of the United States one day. Everyone knows him! In fact, he is more popular than I am! Hell, I grew up here and am thirty-two years older. Funny, right?

He does not like to get in trouble or be called out by anyone in a negative way. If he does, he shuts down, big crocodile tears well-up in his eyes, and he absolutely hates having people see him cry. So this is my only saving grace to get him to calm down and not be so grown up.

Things come easy and naturally to him. He gets the parts in the plays, picked to speak to an astronaut at NASA, always chosen to be an example to the class, things that his brothers rarely get to experience. Maguire enjoys school a lot and loves his friends. He does, however, prefer to hang out with older kids, so socializing has been difficult for us.

A natural athlete is another attribute. I thought, *Cool! I get one out of three!* There isn't a sport he can't master and nothing he doesn't excel at. Playing on all-star baseball teams with fourth graders when he was only in second grade, starting off as a pitcher—it's just another day in the life of Maguire. No sweat, he loves it and he loves being with the older boys. Club soccer, swimming, basketball, lacrosse, surfing, snowboarding—if he wants it, he'll do it, and he'll do it well.

Parents have said to me, "Well, of course, Maguire is good at that, he has two older brothers." However, the truth is, his brothers don't do any of these things. Maguire is just Maguire. He is his own person. So much so, I let him dress how he wants and dye his hair all sorts of colors. I get some judgmental looks and comments from other parents, but this is my kid. I want all my kids to express who they are and be proud of that. I draw the line on getting a tattoo, though. (Smile)

Some challenges we deal with because Maguire is advanced beyond his years is arranging "playdates" with kids his age. This has always been a challenge. He gets bored easily and wants to do things the older boys are doing. For example, he wanted to have a paintball party for his fifth birthday. Yes, you heard me.

He couldn't understand why none of his classmates would come and the parents, well, they would all think I was insane if I indulged him that request.

He is obsessed with being strong, protecting himself and his brothers. He has pellet guns that we take camping (only with Dad) and likes to collect pocket knives (which are all supervised).

> **HE IS OBSESSED WITH BEING STRONG, PROTECTING HIMSELF AND HIS BROTHERS.**

Not only did he want to play with older "toys," he understands adult conversation and likes to learn as much as he can about anything of interest.

He has a tendency to hang out with Caden's peers, who are two grades above him. But when we go on family trips, he gravitates to even older kids.

I am thankful that I have an amazing relationship with Maguire, because he trusts me. He tells me everything that goes on, and he is not a liar. With that said, he has told me about a lot of conversations he has witnessed and that are surely not appropriate for any kid, let alone an eight-year-old. I always use this as a teaching opportunity, and we have long talks about it.

Maguire has a good head on his shoulders, and I trust him. We are still figuring out all this social interaction, and I'm glad that he doesn't have a ton of free time with his sports and other activities.

His brothers' opinion of this third child of mine, this "golden child" in our household, is a whole different story. When you have a younger brother who can do it all, it brings about much disdain. It is not lost on them that Maguire is for all intents and purposes considered smarter, quicker, more popular, braver, funnier than they are. The truth is that he runs circles around his brothers. However, all Maguire wants is acceptance from them, and he gets none. Zero!

He wants to play with them, but they have nothing in common. Kyle is a Lego kid who plays with character figures and uses his imagination. Caden does the same with whatever he is into at the time. He loves Grossery Gang and South Park. He plays with his Plushies. Maguire wants to shoot hoops and ride bikes, something that holds no interest for the others. Maguire never played with "typical" toys. He skipped over all the "kid" stuff.

"My little 'Bother'" is what they call him. He is annoying to them. Thus, because he gets shooed away all the time by his siblings, he figures bugging them and getting negative attention is at least attention. This has caused so much chaos in our house. There are times that they do get along, and it is getting better as they grow older and have more of an understanding for one another.

Maguire begged to start seeing a therapist, just like his brothers. At first, I thought, *You have to be kidding.* However, it actually seemed like a good idea. The therapist's evaluation and description said he was "a fifteen-year-old trapped in an eight-year-old body." The social stuff, connecting with his brothers, and his perfectionism was plenty for them to work on, and it has been great.

It made me feel so validated when the therapist made reference to "kids like Maguire." She has had a few—kids who are so charismatic and wise beyond their years that if their energy is not funneled and they aren't stimulated, they get bored. As I have seen firsthand, this can lead to trouble.

When his brothers are zoning out on video games or whatever has captivated their attention, Maguire has been known to be on a ladder retrieving old toys and balls that have been thrown up on our roof. Another time he was out in the yard with a hammer, hitting pieces of our flagstone. Well, that turned into a costly problem, so we got him a smash box that had a bunch of stuff inside he could crush.

His toys, like I said, are not those of a normal kid his age. Besides his pellet guns, he has a bow and arrow for which he sets up and shoots targets in our backyard. Naturally, he is really good. In fact, he has always said more than once he wants to be a sniper, Navy Seal, big strong brave man. I put him in Tae Kwon Do, but he wants to do MMA and boxing. He thinks that if he needs to protect someone, those are the skills he needs. Maguire, the protector.

Sometimes it may seem that he is embarrassed by his brothers, which is probably partially true. However, the real reason he feels the need to defend is that he doesn't want anyone making fun of them. Kyle will put on his face masks and ride in the car, and Maguire gets so upset. "Kyle, take off that mask! It's so stupid," he'll shout. He literally will get tears in his eyes.

Yes, he probably does look a little strange being a twelve-year-old, wearing a superhero mask just because, and Maguire instinctively knows even as the younger brother that it is not "age appropriate." He is really only wanting to protect his brother. He knows other kids will judge and make fun of him.

Since he was little, he has always "helped" Caden. He would do things for him or tell him how to do things right, he would correct him and make sure he was appropriate and followed the rules at school. Maguire has tackled and taken down an older boy at the beach when he started making fun of Caden. (Disclaimer: We knew this boy, and his parents witnessed the event. The boy deserved a little face in the sand.) The brother bond is stronger than we see, it is unspoken.

THE BROTHER BOND IS STRONGER THAN WE SEE, IT IS UNSPOKEN.

When Caden was younger, he didn't mind so much but as he has gotten older, it has caused conflicts.

"Good job, Caden. How was therapy, Caden? Did you learn how to take turns?" He uses a voice like a teacher, which ends up sounding condescending. It is all coming from a pure place of love. Again, Maguire was born into therapy; it is all he knows.

We finally turned a new page, and Maguire is conscious to let Caden be his big brother (sometimes) and teach him things. It has made their relationship so much better. Maguire has learned to be more patient, because he is aware of what is going on, that he is "letting" Caden teach him.

So you can see, it is a difficult dynamic to say the least. Maguire is used to being the talker of the family, stealing the show, because Kyle and Caden could care less about sharing, or are too zoned out on their electronics. But things are changing, and I am trying to help my boys understand one another and realize how lucky they are to have one another.

Having built-in best friends is pretty amazing. Kyle, being the oldest, tends to not want to be bothered by anyone. He can be mean at times, especially to Maguire. "You ruined my life, things are so much better when you aren't here." Yes, Maguire can cause some crazy in our house, but so can the others, and these comments are so hurtful.

I tell Kyle, "When you get older, do you want Maguire telling people that his older brother is an asshole, or that his older brother is one of his best friends and the coolest?" It puts the situation in perspective, because Kyle wants acceptance from his little brother, too. They all want to be loved, just like we do.

Maguire is gaining more understanding of his brothers and of their differences. Standing on stage this past year alongside his brother when he ran for president of his school was a moment he won't forget. Walking off stage with tears in his eyes, with a feeling that he rarely experienced for Caden—*pride*! He was so proud of his brother, and it was a big turning point for their relationship.

Maguire is understanding, slowly, that he has to share the spotlight, that there are two other golden children in this family. Maguire will always be "that kid," but he knows his role is more than that of boy wonder. He is here to be the younger brother of Caden who has Autism and Kyle who has ADHD Inattentive. He is here to help spread the word that different is *awesome*, and dying his hair, wearing his own style, being who he truly is—owning it—is his own form of awesome.

> MAGUIRE WILL ALWAYS BE "THAT KID," BUT HE KNOWS HIS ROLE IS MORE THAN THAT OF BOY WONDER.

TEN

MY BROTHER CADEN

My name is Maguire, and I am nine years old. I am Caden's little brother. I am going to tell you what it is like having a brother with Autism. Being Caden's little brother is cool, but sometimes it can be hard, and just because he has Autism doesn't change him—he is a person, too.

If you don't know what Autism is, I will tell you about it. Autism is a thing you are born with. Some people have mild Autism and some people have severe Autism. Autism can be a lot of things. Do you know what ADHD is? What about ADD or Sensory Processing Disorder? These are all things people with Autism can have. My brother Caden has major sensory issues.

I always thought Caden just dressed funny. He loves wearing beanies. He wears them almost every single day, even when it is hot out. When Caden wears hats or beanies, it doesn't bother me, it's just my brother. But some people think he's weird and stare. I don't like when people stare at him. I get very protective of him sometimes. I often wonder if it bothers him, or if he even knows people think he is weird? Also, Caden loves blankets. He likes fuzzy soft blankets and blankets that weigh a lot. He has one on his bed that is 20 pounds! He likes to walk in our backyard listening to music with his headphones

> **I OFTEN WONDER IF IT BOTHERS HIM, OR IF HE EVEN KNOWS PEOPLE THINK HE IS WEIRD?**

and paces back and forth. My friends come over and wonder what he is doing. I just say, "That's just what Caden does." I don't think I have ever thought about what it is like to be in his head.

In 2010, I was born, and Caden was already diagnosed with Autism. Since I was a little baby, I would go everywhere with my mom, and my mom was the person who took Caden to therapy. My mom used to say that I was going to be so smart from absorbing all the therapy going on around me. I thought therapy was just normal, because that is what we did. When I was growing up, I always wanted to do the therapies Caden did. He got to play and there were always teachers coming to our house to spend time with him. Whenever I wanted to join in, Caden would get mad at me and never let me. My mom would tell me this was Caden's time, and it wasn't fun play time for him, it was hard work. It was still hard for me to not want to do what they were doing. There was a part of me that wanted to be just like my brother.

Sometimes I am more of an older brother than a younger one. I have helped Caden with his homework, taught him if he has done something wrong, and stood up for him if anyone is bullying him.

Even though Caden has Autism, he is always caring, nice, funny, and everyone wants to be his friend. He is never mean (except to me, but I know it's because that is what brothers do). He is into different things, like old video games—his favorite is Cup Head—and gets on the computer and finds the coolest videos.

> EVEN THOUGH CADEN HAS AUTISM, HE IS ALWAYS CARING, NICE, FUNNY, AND EVERYONE WANTS TO BE HIS FRIEND.

I am proud of Caden, because when things are hard for him, he never gives up and always pushes through. I am very lucky to have Caden as my big brother. He has taught me that, even though life can be hard, I can do anything if I try.

ELEVEN

CADEN FOR PRESIDENT

A life rule I've had since the beginning: One foot in front of the other, live day by day, and never worry about the future. This has proven to be a rule that is hard to follow. Especially with having a kid with Autism. Being on the "spectrum" is just that, a spectrum. An Autism diagnosis is extremely broad, and there are so many learning disorders that fall under this umbrella. When Caden received this diagnosis at the age of two, we were left with an unknown future. We didn't know what we were looking at long term, so eventually we realized it did not help to worry about something we had no control over—the future. We have always tried to stay in the present.

I read one book when Caden was diagnosed. ONE. That was all it took for me to go back to my non-reading ways. If I had believed what I read, I don't know if I would have been able to live the life I have. I definitely would have frequented the bars more, cocktailing it up, my hair would be thin and grey, and I would be a complete mess. Perhaps I would have turned into "that mom" I always had nightmares about—the caricature one who had all boys and was haggard with her bottle of booze and smoking a cigarette, looking older than her own mother.

Would I believe that Caden wouldn't graduate high school, go to college, or hold a job? He wouldn't get married or even have a girlfriend. Friends, forget about it—he would live in solitude indefinitely. He would live in my house forever, and I would have a pretend relationship with him, always wondering if I was getting through and if we really connected. Could you imagine being a parent of a newly diagnosed toddler, believing all of this? Pretty depressing.

As I write this, we are in the beginning of Caden's last year at elementary school, and things are starting to get REAL. I remember when he was in kindergarten, thinking that we had so much time ahead of us before I really needed to start worrying about things. Focusing on holding his pencil correctly and using scissors was so much easier than being concerned whether he was at the right reading level and if his friends would leave him in the dust when he went to middle school. Nonetheless, the time is here, and as much as I don't want to think about the future, I have to.

Caden has blown my mind and exceeded my every expectation! He touches the hearts of everyone he meets, and his circle of peers surrounded him for the past six years, giving him support and the courage to be himself. He is no longer the little boy who would sit in his car seat, silent behind me, not responding to my questions. He is opinionated and knows what he likes. Caden has a say in everything we do and doesn't let anyone push him around or tell him what to do. He can do it, he's "got this," and he wants to make sure everyone knows he's not an "idiot"—these are his own words, not mine.

> **WHEN YOU JUDGE SOMEONE BASED ON A DIAGNOSIS, YOU MISS OUT ON THAT PERSON'S ABILITIES, BEAUTY, AND UNIQUENESS.**

I find myself once again, having to make the decision of which path to take with middle school approaching quickly. Although very similar to his older brother, Caden is also very different, and our concerns for middle school are different. Caden has a core group of buddies he is really connected to. Heading into a huge public middle school next year can be intimidating to anyone, and he's starting at the bottom of the totem pole. Finding your place, routine, new schedule, and "rules," like where you sit for lunch and who your friends are, are all enough to cause anxiety. There is so much to adapt to, it is survival mode with each kid fending for themselves. My fear is that Caden would be left in the dust. I try not to step in, I let Caden navigate his days with friends and school, but this is a life-changing decision that I need to make for him as his parent. If we decide to send him to the neighborhood school, this is just what happens—kids are trying to find their own way.

Kyle, my oldest is emotional, sensitive, and borders depression, so attending a large middle school would have devastated him. Caden, however, is a happy-go-lucky kid. He is who he is with no care what others think. He loves his friends, but wouldn't take it personally if they weren't around as much, or even be aware, which means he would end up hanging out by himself all day. The social aspect and mental well-being of my children trumps academics. They can always learn math, reading, and writing, but if they are ruined inside, what good is math going to do them? Giving my children the self-confidence and safe, supportive environment to be who they are and to discover their strengths is my main concern.

> CADEN IS A HAPPY-GO-LUCKY KID. HE IS WHO HE IS WITH NO CARE WHAT OTHERS THINK.

We are in the application process for Caden to become a "Husky" (school mascot) and join his older brother at private school. This school has changed not only Kyle's life, but all of ours as a family. I know it will be a life changer for Caden as well. I sit with anxious, excited feelings, knowing what it has already done for Kyle. The possibilities for Caden to grow are endless. He had his interview last week. I was nervous, actually scared. This letting go and believing in Caden 100 percent was new for me.

He's just gotten through his elementary school presidency campaign, where he lost by two votes. He blew not only me, but every single other parent and kid, out of the water with his speech. He does have something to say. That was a *huge* step for us all. Now this interview. The same nervous feelings and thoughts were all coming back: *Please don't do anything funny or embarrassing. Please sit still and answer the questions appropriately, and please just be you.* I had told Caden that this was important, it was him not talking to a therapist, but a teacher, so act appropriately. I wanted him to be on his best behavior, but I wanted them to see Caden for who he is, because that is the best part.

Caden came out of the room when his interview was done. It was our turn. Tome and I sat on the couch and started our conversation with the head of admissions. Luckily, being Kyle's mom, they know me because I have been very involved in the school. Not only was this a bonus, but it made the conversation more comfortable and our nerves were calmed. Mrs. B shared with us her conversation with Caden and the questions and answers they went over. He knew he was there to decide if he wanted to come to this school next year or not. He made comments about liking the art in the office and was very comfortable. He did have a hard time sitting still, which we explained was due to his sensory processing. At the end, she asked Caden if he had any questions. Of course he did. "If you had a transgender dog, what would you name it?" That was his question. I am sure this came from some YouTube video he had seen, and that is what he wanted to know. Mrs. B told him, "Spencer." One of the many amazing reasons we love this school is that it is the real world. There is no box to fit in, and the kids beam with originality. There is a full on raver kid at the school, plastic backpack, lollipop, and all. Kids who are open about their sexual identity, and kids like my son Kyle who still dresses in his superhero costume (although I think that phase is over). Point being, the question was not that shocking.

I have learned through the years to put positive energy out into the world. If you believe and have faith, amazing things can happen. Open the doors and allow light to shine on your path. I can sit worrying and allow my anxious thoughts to get the best of me, wondering if Caden will be accepted into private school. Or I can also choose to believe and know in my heart, big things are about to happen. He will get accepted, and he will amaze us all once again with his special gifts.

Sometimes I catch myself worrying too much about what is socially acceptable for him to be doing. Caden likes to pace back and forth—we call him the lion in the cage. He needs this, it is an outlet, his time out after working so hard and exerting energy to maintain focus in the classroom. He knows the times when he needs to be alone and just be in his zone. He is listening to his body. I had thought for a minute about working on this behavior, but then realized, he would replace it with something else. And who cares if he is walking back and forth? It isn't all the time, and in twenty years when he is making millions being a world-renowned scientist, no one will pay attention to his pacing. My husband loves the story of when Caden was in pre-school. We were there for an afterschool program to watch them compete in their own Olympics. Caden was walking in circles. His teacher said, "Caden, stop walking in circles." He looked at her and asked, "Should I walk in a square instead?" That pretty much sums up Caden.

The amount of gratitude I have every day for the amazing gift I have been given with all of my children, but especially Caden and his Autism, is immeasurable. It is a gift I didn't see for a long time, and now I am embracing. I hear more often than I would like that I have my hands full, and people express surprise that I do all the things I do. I know I have a lot on my plate, but that is part of being a mom. We bring these amazing lives into the world, and we have no idea what we are going to get.

> IT IS A GIFT I DIDN'T SEE FOR A LONG TIME, AND NOW I AM EMBRACING.

Each day we turn a new page in their book of life, discovering something new. I don't find myself looking at other families as perfect or feeling sorry for myself, assuming that they have it easier. No one's life is easy. Society pushes the image that we all should have a picture-perfect life, but we know that is far from the truth. I can assume all I want, but the family that looks totally pulled together has its own issues, too.

Autism has changed my life. I am a better person because of it. I have gone through several frustrating moments and stressful, anxious days. At times I felt like I was the worst mother. But I am not the worst mother, I am an awesome mom, and Autism has made me the best mom. We all have hope and big dreams for our children. We want them to explore the world and find happiness and love. We want all their dreams to come true.

Having a child with Autism gives hope a whole different meaning. I have hope for things that I don't know will ever be obtainable. I hope Caden has an amazing time during his school years, experiencing friendships that will last a lifetime. I hope he goes to dances and football games and finds a club or sport he loves. I hope he discovers a passion for art or music and sticks with it, inspired by his teachers. I hope he keeps up academically with his peers and shows others how smart he is. I hope he goes to a college of his choice and parties his ass off like I did… or not. I hope he finds his path and discovers who he is. I hope he knows he is great and sees what I have seen

> **BECAUSE OF YOU, I SEE THINGS THROUGH DIFFERENT EYES.**

in him since he was born. I hope he experiences true love, gets married, and has a family of his own. I hope I get to see his face full of happiness and pride when he has children of his own, and he realizes that all I ever wanted was for him to be happy. I hope he knows how much I love him. I hope for it all.

I don't know what tomorrow will bring, and I don't know if all my dreams for my children will come true. I do know that Caden is about to take on the world. Doors are about to open and what lies on the other side is going to be magic. I can't imagine being much prouder than I already am, but I know it is going to happen. For years, I wanted to get a tattoo that represented how I live life and how my kids live life. It took me years of not looking, knowing it would come to me when it was the right time. About a year ago, I found it.

"Sisu." The definition: extraordinary determination, courage and resoluteness in the face of extreme adversity. An action mindset that enables individuals to see beyond their present limitations and into what might be. Taking action against the odds and reaching beyond observed capacities. A universal capacity for which the potential exists within all individuals.

Every time I see this word on my arm, it reminds me of my strength and determination. It reminds me that I am human and anything is possible. There are no limitations to what I can do or what my kids can do, and no one can take that away. I will continue to believe and wake up every day grateful for a new day. I will smile and allow myself to be great. If I am great, my boys will be even greater.

The best part of my day is when I call his name, "Caden?"

He replies, "What, you love me, don't you?"

Yes I do! My relationship with Caden is evolving every day. I no longer have to hope for a giggle, smile, or glance for me to feel connected to him. I *see* him, deep in his eyes full of life, and he is ready to break out of his shell. He has an enormous heart and capacity for empathy beyond what we see. His emotions are deep, and he has a hard time allowing himself to feel sad. He has a hard time understanding that he can be both happy and sad. If he is sad, he can't be happy, so he rarely lets himself tap into deep emotions.

He sent me an emoji text message one day. It was simply three characters—a book, a wedding ring, and a coffin. I knew instantly what it meant. He is fearful and sad of the unknown. He is scared to go away to college and leave everything he knows behind, especially me who has been his constant his entire life. He is afraid of marriage and death. He thinks about these things often, and they sit deep inside. In the past year, I have made it a point to talk to Caden, to sit down with him and take his phone away so I have his full attention.

I want to be a part of his life, I want to know him. I want him to share with me all that he holds inside. Just

> **HE IS FEARFUL AND SAD OF THE UNKNOWN.**

because he doesn't ask, doesn't mean he isn't curious about what is "wrong" with him, or why he is different. Just because he doesn't come home from school and tell me about his day, doesn't mean he doesn't have something to say. Usually parents are sick of hearing their kids talk and want a minute of peace and quiet. I seek out conversation and want to know what is going on inside that head. It is going to take time, and I know for now, I have to be proactive if I want to have a connection with Caden. He no longer is the forgotten son, the one who stays behind, because we think he wants to be alone.

 I have taken Kyle and Maguire on mother-son weekends with their friends. Caden has always been the forgotten one, because I believed he didn't want to go. "Mom, when do I get to go somewhere with you alone?" This question hit me right in the face. Why did I ever assume he didn't want to do something special with me, just like his brothers? I am so looking forward to our special time together, and I can't wait to see what he comes up with and where he wants to go. I think I am more excited than he is to spend some alone time and really get to know my son.

TWELVE

I'M THE BIG BROTHER

Being Caden's brother can be fun and strange. It's definitely strange with the way he talks. He talks about things that I don't know about, and sometimes in a strange voice. It is also really fun to hang out with him, because he has a very good imagination and always thinks of things we can do. Maybe because we are really close, it makes us get along really well. He never avoids me, he always wants me to hang out with him and do a bunch of stuff he wants me to do.

THE HARD THINGS

Being a big brother, you have to be supportive, even if those choices aren't that good. Because Caden has Autism, it makes it weird to hang out with him sometimes. He says random things when I am around and it makes it a little bit awkward. He does things sometimes that are not appropriate or allowed. He could say something inappropriate to someone that he doesn't even know. This is embarrassing, and I feel like he is not able to go out in public. Because we are really close in age, it makes me feel like he is not responsible enough to do certain things. When he does things, people might make fun of him, and it would make him sad. I am protective of my brother. I do not want to see him get in trouble or upset. We don't really have a lot in common. He likes Plants vs Zombies and inappropriate stuff like South Park. Me, I like superheroes and…

> **I AM PROTECTIVE OF MY BROTHER. I DO NOT WANT TO SEE HIM GET IN TROUBLE OR UPSET.**

THE GOOD THINGS

Caden and I get along really well. Most likely because we are a little over a year apart. Caden is a super fun kid with a sense of humor who happens to be my brother. Even though he is not that interactive with his friends, he does play with me. Caden is almost never mean to me. He tells me about all these cool new toys and things he learns about before I know about them. If we could, I would find a game that we both like, and we could play together. Caden always thinks ahead and never asks people what he should be doing. He just does what he is supposed to do.

Caden is really caring. He doesn't like to see people get into trouble. When he sees others get in trouble, he feels bad—he always tries to help them do what they are supposed to do, so they won't get into trouble. He has such a big heart, and he is always helping. He never says "*later*," he always does things when he is told. He also cares about our animals, asking me to feed my reptiles because he knows they are hungry and doesn't want them to starve. Caden is creative. He makes the funniest videos. He doesn't want to share them, but I still watch them on his recorder and they are really funny. He may come across shy, but he really isn't.

Even though he has Autism, that's what makes Caden, Caden. He has different learning skills, and I am really proud of him for making it through elementary school, because it was really hard for me.

> EVEN THOUGH HE HAS AUTISM, THAT'S WHAT MAKES CADEN, CADEN.

Caden likes to be by himself, and I really don't get it. He is this funny kid who knows how to interact with me, but doesn't interact with others. The kids at school all really like him and want to hang out with him. He is starting to make friends, which is cool.

Caden, I am so lucky to have you as a brother. We have been together for our entire lives, and you are a good person with a good heart. You just need to start believing in yourself. Having you as my brother has made my life exciting. I always have so much fun with you, and you make me laugh. We hang out all the time, and I guess you are like my best friend. I love you.

> **I ALWAYS HAVE SO MUCH FUN WITH YOU, AND YOU MAKE ME LAUGH.**

THIRTEEN

TURNING POINT

The day Caden was diagnosed, we knew the next step was jumping into intensive ABA therapy. It was going to become our life. We would completely immerse ourselves in this new world. Our minutes, hours, and days were filled with rotating therapists showing up at our door, sometimes greeted with a smile and others with a cry. Caden was a working machine, it became his norm and now is all he knows. Of all my boys, he is my most compliant.

I was trying to juggle a four-year-old and my ever-growing tummy, pregnant with my third boy. My life was chaos, and there was never a moment of peace. We were in the middle of a major remodel (because we needed to throw that in the mix) and were living in a small rental in Hermosa Beach. An original beach home, a classic. Plumbing issues and a lack of storage and space, appliances that didn't work properly, and a backyard, a jungle, that had been growing for decades. But we were happy. Every day, Caden's smile would melt my heart, and Kyle was the best big brother, trying to teach him all he knew. Tome would come home from work and, although I was exhausted, I couldn't wait to share with him what Caden had been working on that day.

> EVERY DAY, CADEN'S SMILE WOULD MELT MY HEART, AND KYLE WAS THE BEST BIG BROTHER, TRYING TO TEACH HIM ALL HE KNEW.

There are so many things I have forgotten from the past. Obstacles that were overcome and struggles that I didn't remember being a reality for Caden. Tome would always tell me that his first suspicion that Caden had Autism was his lack of speech. I didn't remember it that way. I knew he pulled on me all the time and would point to things. His speech was definitely delayed, but I didn't remember it the way Tome did. It wasn't until I started journaling, writing for me, to get in touch and acknowledge my feelings, that I began to reflect on the past. I was moving too quickly to slow down and see the journey we had been on.

Memories flooded my head and tears welled up in my eyes. I wasn't used to crying or feeling my emotions, this was all new to me. I was pulling up all my old photos and videos off the computer, spending hours laughing and crying. I was in awe, how could I forget about these moments of time that were so crucial and important? I wasn't holding space, and I didn't have the capacity at the time to fully embrace what was happening. How could I? I was a soon-to-be-mom of three, a wife, a house cleaner, a cook, a taxi driver, and a dog walker, and I was trying to work a "real job," because all that other stuff doesn't pay. Women are real life superheroes, no doubt.

 I sat and watched videos that we had taken on our flip recorder, which totally sucks. The sound and picture quality are so bad, it is amazing what our phones can do today. I am standing in our kitchen with Caden in my arms, legs around my waist. We are looking eye to eye. I say "ready, set," and pause.

 "GO," Caden yells, and I fling him down through my legs like a sack of potatoes. He laughs uncontrollably, feeling every sensation in his sensory-seeking, two-year-old body. I ask if he wants to do it again. We do this over and over. I sat and watched the video with tears running down my face. I had a flutter in my stomach. I remembered that moment and the feelings I had that day. It was the biggest accomplishment for him to say "go." I cried and I cried. I had forgotten how far this little guy had come. I was in this fast-paced hamster wheel putting one foot in front of the other, never looking back. I was living in the moment, focusing on the now, and the goals we were working on. I had forgotten how much we celebrated "go." My tears were of joy, gratitude, and overwhelming pride for Caden.

As the days passed and the therapy sessions continued, I decided to get Caden tested, a full neuropsychic evaluation. He was still only two, but I wanted to know from a professional exactly what was going on with him. Based on a thirty-minute observation in a small room, Caden was diagnosed at our Regional Center. Although I was thankful for the diagnosis, I really didn't care about anything else they had to say. I was referred to a reputable psychologist out in San Fernando Valley, Dr. Mary Large. After asking my grandfather for $5,000 to pay for the testing, we scheduled our appointment.

The day arrived for our first testing date. I now had a new baby, baby number three. I dropped Kyle at preschool, packed Caden and Maguire into the car, and headed out to the Valley for the day. The testing lasted four straight days. I didn't know if Caden could handle it. The doctor was very nice and explained what would be taking place during the testing time. She explained to me that she would be looking at all his deficits and pointing out all the negatives. I looked at her and kind of nodded my head. She said, "I tell this to all my parents when they come in, and as the testing occurs, everyone is always caught off guard when I point out things, even though they are

> MY TEARS WERE OF JOY, GRATITUDE, AND OVERWHELMING PRIDE FOR CADEN.

warned." She continued to explain that it was great if Caden could clap his hands or sing "Happy Birthday," but she needed to see what he couldn't do. It made sense, and I understood. Each day as the testing continued, Caden would do various tasks, and I could see her shaking her head and jotting things down. She had him pull a little duck behind him on a string. She wanted him to walk backward, pulling the duck. He did at first, but then turned around and ran. That was "wrong." Each time she marked something down, my heart sank. She warned me, but it still happened. I don't think anyone wants to hear all the "bad" things about their kids, they want to hear how amazing and wonderful they are. How could this adorable, brown-eyed toddler with the biggest dimples be anything but amazing and wonderful?

> "THERE IS NO GREATER DISABILITY IN SOCIETY THAN THE INABILITY TO SEE A PERSON AS MORE."
>
> —ROBERT M. HENSEL

The test ended and the doctor told me it would take her a few weeks to complete the report. It is very detailed and long. I was just happy that I didn't have to drive out to the Valley one more day and that Caden could go back to his normal therapy routine.

My house was full with joy and laughter and the sounds of a new baby. We were now getting settled in our new home. Caden continued to work with his therapists each and every day. I watched how hard he worked and wished I could do it all for him. I sat in my kitchen one day, baby asleep and having two seconds to catch up on work. My phone rang.

"Hi, this is Dr. Large. I am done with your report. I wanted to call you and chat before I sent it to you in the mail."

My heart was racing. I left the last day of testing without thinking one moment about the results and what could come of this. I knew I didn't have any control over it, so I did what I do best and kept busy.

She continued, "I just want to tell you that you have one remarkable little boy." I lost it. Every tear I had held in since Caden's diagnosis came out that moment. I sat and cried, and I couldn't stop. She told me that in nine months' time, Caden had gained two years of knowledge. He was closing the gap. It was the best news I had ever received from anyone in my whole life. I had been going at the speed of light since the day of his diagnosis. I never looked back, never took a second to do anything else, and put every ounce of myself into helping him. But I didn't know what I was doing. I was putting so much faith into something I didn't know if it was working or not, but I had no choice but to keep moving forward. This phone call, these words that were spoken, gave me affirmation that I was doing the right thing. That all my energy, effort, time, love, and perseverance was all for something. My little boy was kicking ass!

In my journey of self-discovery, I have had to take a deep look inside. I have had challenges to overcome. I have faced my fears and continue to face them, knowing that is the only way change will happen. I have been asked what event or thing in my life was my aha moment, the moment that changed my life. So many assume it was the day Caden received his diagnosis. This was a day that gave me direction, a path to go down, a starting point. The day I received that phone call from Dr. Large, that was my turning point, that was the beginning of my life with Autism.

> I HAVE FACED MY FEARS AND CONTINUE TO FACE THEM, KNOWING THAT IS THE ONLY WAY CHANGE WILL HAPPEN.

FOURTEEN

HOPE & LOVE

The one thing that has been a constant on this journey is hope. Hope is the light at the end of the tunnel. Sometimes that light is hard to see, but I know it is there. Even in my darkest moments, I know that the light will soon shine. Hope is what keeps me going, hope is what gives me the courage to face my toughest days. Hope is energy, hope is life, hope is something bigger than me, something I cannot see. Hope is what will strengthen you as you face what lies ahead, so don't ever lose hope!

There are so many unknowns in life, with raising kids, and especially raising kids with special needs. There are uncertainties and sometimes we feel out of control. Sometimes we can feel lost and confused and all alone, like our world is caving in. Make the choice to wake up each day feeling blessed for what you have been given. Grab hold of the day and decide how you want to face the challenges that may come your way. We can't control what happens each day, but we can choose how we react.

My son asked me today what the best part of our family was. "The best part is I love everyone! I love you, I love Dad, I love Kyle, I love Maguire." As my heart melted, I told him I think he is the best part of our family, because he reminds me every day that we have love. I am loved. My family is loved.

> I THINK HE IS THE BEST PART OF OUR FAMILY, BECAUSE HE REMINDS ME EVERY DAY THAT WE HAVE LOVE.

So, when you are having moments of sadness or feel like nothing is going right, or you don't know what tomorrow will bring, remember that you are not alone. Remember your village and that you are loved. And know that no matter what, you will get through the day with HOPE & LOVE.

GLOSSARY

Applied Behavior Analysis (ABA)
A type of therapy that is based on the science of learning and behavior. ABA therapy applies our understanding of how behavior works to real situations. The goal is to increase behaviors that are helpful and decrease behaviors that are harmful or affect learning.

Attention-Deficit Hyperactivity Disorder (ADHD)
A neurobehavioral condition that interferes with a person's ability to pay attention and exercise age-appropriate inhibition

Autism Spectrum Disorder (ASD)
Autism is a neurological and developmental disorder that begins early in childhood and can last through a person's life. It affects how a person acts and interacts with others, communicates, and learns. It includes what used to be known as Asperger's syndrome and pervasive developmental disorders.

It is called a "spectrum" disorder because people with ASD can have a range of symptoms. People with ASD might have problems talking with others, or they might not look people in the eye when people are talking to them. They may also have restricted interests and repetitive behaviors. They may spend a lot of time putting things in order, or they may say the same sentence again and again. They may often seem to be in their "own world."

It is a spectrum. An entire rainbow. It is hard to just say, "My kid is Autistic," because what does that mean? It can mean a lot of things.

Candida

Here is the scientific meaning: Candidiasis refers to an overgrowth of the yeast Candida. *Leaky gut* is a more serious consequence, occurring when Candida causes the intestinal wall to become permeable and allows partially digested proteins and other toxins to be released into the body. To cleanse the body of Candida, eliminate sugar, flour, and dairy.

Cannabidiol (CBD)

CBD is a cannabis compound that has significant medical benefits, but does not make people feel "stoned" and can actually counteract the psychoactivity of THC (Tetrahydrocannabinol, the chemical largely responsible for marijuana's psychological effects). CBD has helped people with inflammation, pain, anxiety, psychosis, seizures, spasms, focus, insomnia, ... the list goes on and on.

Cognitive Behavior Therapy (CBT)

CBT takes into account the thoughts we have about things, the feelings that result, and the behavior that follows.

Essential Oils

Essential oils are concentrated plant extracts that retain the natural smell and flavor, or "essence," of their source. Essential oils are used for various purposes from health and wellness, to beauty, cooking, spiritual and religious practices, and aromatherapy, to name a few.

Genetically Modified Organisms (GMO)

GMOs are living organisms in which the genetic material has been artificially manipulated in a laboratory through genetic engineering. This creates combinations of plant, animal, bacteria, and viral genes that do not occur in nature or through traditional crossbreeding methods.

Grossery Gang

Little rubber disgusting character toys that are my son's obsession. He has collected them all. What's a mother to do?

Individual Education Programs (IEP)
IEPs help ensure a student with Autism, or any other learning disability, is receiving the best possible services in school. IEPs are based on each student's unique strengths and challenges. They help define a student's personal educational goals and lay out the steps that will be taken to achieve those goals.

Lindamood Bell
An intense reading and comprehension program that teaches kids/adults to learn at their full potential.

Neurofeedback
Neurofeedback, also called *neurotherapy* or *neurobiofeedback*, is a type of biofeedback that uses real-time displays of brain activity—most commonly electro-encephalography—to teach self-regulation of brain function.

NeuroFit
A program created to help neuropathway efficiency with a nonmedical approach. Using movement sequences based on the neurobiological process of brain development, it can improve how the brain receives, and processes information. Increased neuropathway efficiency leads to improved motor, processing, and cognitive function.

NeuroZone

A place where Caden and Kyle received neurofeedback.

    The NeuroZone is a group of dedicated specialists who work with individuals with neurodevelopmental delays, learning disabilities, and behavioral issues. They have one common goal—to provide the most comprehensive neurodevelopment, academic, and behavioral evaluation with a subsequent integrated remediation program for each client.

Occupational Therapy (OT)

Occupational therapy helps people work on cognitive, physical, social, and motor skills. The goal is to improve everyday skills that allow people to become more independent and participate in a wide range of activities. For people with Autism, OT focuses on play skills, learning strategies, and self-care. OT can also help manage sensory issues.

Physical Therapy (PT)

The treatment of disease, injury, or deformity by physical methods such as massage, heat treatment, and exercise rather than by drugs or surgery.

    Specific to kids who have disabilities, PT can help the following:

- Functional development, motor, and mobility skills

- Using exercises to increase strength, endurance, and joint mobility
- Balance and coordination activities
- Increase muscle strength
- Increase coordination

Regional Center
Nonprofit organizations that contract with the Department of Educational Services to provide or coordinate services or support for individuals with developmental disabilities.

Speech Therapy (ST)
Training to help people with speech and language problems to speak more clearly. This is the definition. However, many assume someone with a speech issue has a slur or a lisp or can't pronounce certain letters. Yes, this is part of it, but there is a whole lot more that falls under the speech category.

Speech therapy is an intervention service that focuses on improving a child's speech and ability to understand and express language, including nonverbal language. Speech therapy includes two components: 1) Coordinating the mouth to produce sounds to form words and sentences (to address articulation, fluency, and voice volume regulation); and 2) Understanding and expressing language (to address the use of language through written, pictorial, body, and sign forms, and the use of language through alternative communication systems such as social media, computers, and iPads). In addition, the role of SLPs (speech-language pathologists) in treating swallowing disorders has broadened to include all aspects of feeding.

Student Success Team (SST)
A team of professionals at school (principal, teacher, school psychologist, speech therapist, etc.) that, after observation and testing, develops a plan of action to help the student's success at school.

Tinctures
A tincture is a concentrated liquid herbal extract. It is typically made by soaking herbs and other plant parts in alcohol for weeks to extract the active constituents.

Velcro Shoes—The Stories of My Life
Velcro Shoes is my blog created to share stories that are real, raw, and vulnerable. It is a place to feel safe and to connect with others—to know you are not alone. There is no judgment, only support, compassion, and a place to be heard or listened to. www.Velcro-Shoes.com

RESOURCES

*For support, services, research,
and information related to Autism*

There are numerous organizations, websites, blogs that can provide information, support, and extend the learning about Autism for family members, those who care for them, advocates, and friends who want to learn more. Some of the many national organizations are presented here. We have also listed those that are local to Alli's family, including many that they have used over the years. It is important to note that most states have similar organizations to assist you and your family or friends. We share them here to help those across the county know the breadth of types of organizations that are available to help and support those with Autism and their families and communities.

National Organizations, Websites, Publications, and Blogs

NEXT for Autism • www.nextforautism.org
NEXT for AUTISM transforms the national landscape of services for people with Autism by strategically designing, launching, and supporting innovative

programs. We believe that individuals with Autism have the potential to live fulfilling, productive lives when supported by excellent services and connected to their communities. We continually ask, what's next for people on the Autism spectrum?

Autism Speaks • www.autismspeaks.org
Autism Speaks is dedicated to promoting solutions, across the spectrum and throughout the lifespan, for the needs of individuals with Autism and their families. We do this through advocacy and support; increasing understanding and acceptance of people with Autism; and advancing research into the causes and better interventions for Autism spectrum disorder and related conditions.

Wolf & Friends • www.wolfandfriends.com
Meet like-minded women in your neighborhood who are also raising children with special needs such as Autism, ADHD, learning differences, developmental delays, anxiety, giftedness, behavioral challenges, mental health issues, sensory processing disorders and Down syndrome.

Connect with new friends and mentors—in a private, judgment-free space.

Get access to a curated content feed to read relevant news, shop stylish and developmentally appropriate products, and get lifestyle tips from special needs parents and experts.

RESOURCES

Find developmental and behavioral pediatricians, occupational therapists, speech and language pathologists, behaviorists, psychiatrists, psychologists, art therapists, feeding therapists, social skills therapists, teletherapists, specialized schools, classes, camps, nonprofits and more—by specialty and locations across the United States.

Turning Pointe Autism Foundation • turningpointeautismfoundation.org
Turning Pointe Autism Foundation was founded in 2007 by Kim and Randy Wolf to provide families with the support needed when managing the challenges faced by children with Autism. The Wolfs personally understood this because their son Jack is impacted. With the need growing for services, the Wolfs expanded the Foundation's commitment to incorporate educational initiatives, family supports, residential plans, and recreation programs. Turning Pointe Autism Foundation continues to create innovative programs and services to assist individuals and families as they navigate through the lifelong impact of Autism.

Organization for Autism Research • researchautism.org
The Organization for Autism Research (OAR) was created in December 2001 to apply research to the challenges of Autism. OAR defines applied research as research that directly impacts the day-to-day quality of life of learners with Autism. It entails the systematic

investigation of variables associated with positive outcomes in such areas as education, communication, self-care, social skills, employment, behavior, and adult and community living. OAR funds pilot studies and targeted research within specific modalities and issues affecting the Autism community, primarily for studies whose outcomes offer new insights into the behavioral and social development of individuals with Autism with an emphasis on communications, education, and vocational challenges. OAR's programs revolve around funding new research and disseminating evidence-based information.

The Autism Community in Action • tacanow.org

The Autism Community in Action (TACA), formerly Talk About Curing Autism, is a U.S. based nonprofit. **Mission statement**: TACA provides education, support, and hope to families living with Autism. **Vision statement**: For every individual diagnosed with Autism to lead an independent life.

The Autism Research Institute • www.autism.org

The Autism Research Institute (ARI) is the hub of a worldwide network of parents and professionals concerned with Autism. ARI was founded in 1967 to conduct and foster scientific research designed to improve the methods of diagnosing, treating, and preventing Autism. ARI also disseminates research findings to parents and others worldwide seeking help. The ARI

RESOURCES

data bank, the world's largest, contains over 42,000 detailed case histories of Autistic children from over 60 countries. ARI publishes the *Autism Research Review International*, a quarterly newsletter covering biomedical and educational advances in autism research.

The Doug Flutie Jr. Foundation for Autism • www.flutiefoundation.org
The Doug Flutie Jr. Foundation for Autism's goal is to help families affected by Autism live life to the fullest. Through our grant programs and partnerships, we help people with Autism get access to care, lead active lifestyles and grow toward adult independence. Our programs and activities improve the quality of everyday life for people and families affected by Autism along **seven key dimensions** that are critical to living each day fully. We aim to provide a path for education and/or employment during the day; opportunities for physical and social activity outside of work/school; and the tools to be safe, supported, and informed at all times.

The Asperger/Autism Network • www.aane.org
The Asperger/Autism Network (AANE) works with individuals, families, and professionals to help people with Asperger Syndrome and similar Autism spectrum profiles build meaningful, connected lives. We do this by providing information, education, community, support, and advocacy, all in an atmosphere of validation and respect. While our primary mission

is to assist individuals affected by AS, AANE is an inclusive organization that also serves people who have other neurological differences or who feel our services would be helpful. Individuals do not need to have a professional diagnosis of Asperger Syndrome in order to benefit from AANE's services. In addition to the services we provide from our home base, AANE works in close partnership with other Asperger's and Autism organizations throughout New England, as well as disability organizations that offer services relevant to the Autism population.

Southwest Autism Research & Resource Center • www.autismcenter.org
Established in 1997, the Southwest Autism Research & Resource Center's (SARRC) mission is to advance research and provide a lifetime of support for individuals with Autism and their families.

SARRC provides programs that address the needs of individuals with Autism spectrum disorder (ASD) of all ages by offering an early intervention program for newly diagnosed children up to six years of age; an eight-classroom inclusive preschool for children from eighteen months to five years of age; K-12 school consultation services; home-based programs; intensive parent training for families living in rural communities; community-based life skills and vocational experiences for teens (ages 13-18); and employment services for adults.

RESOURCES

In 2018, SARRC served 1,014 children, teens, and adults with ASD through our clinical and research programs; educated 6,650 parents, family members, typical peers, and community members; and provided training to 575 educational and medical professionals.

Lindamood-Bell • www.lindamoodbell.com
Lindamood-Bell has pioneered programs to develop the sensory-cognitive processes that underlie reading and comprehension.

Best Day Foundation • www.bestdayfoundation.org
Best Day Foundation enables children and young adults with special needs to build confidence and self-esteem through adventure activities that stretch their limits, expand their true potential, reinforce their achievement, and connect them with diverse populations in their community.

National Ability Center • discovernac.org
The National Ability Center empowers individuals of all abilities by building self-esteem, confidence, and lifetime skills through sports, recreation, and educational programs.

We are the seekers and explorers, the fun-makers and adventurers. We believe life doesn't stop unfolding just because we have a (dis)ability. We're adaptive. Our NAC family draws from decades of experience working with people of all abilities, harnessing the power of specialized equipment, techniques, teaching methods and over 1,900 volunteers.

Autism Parenting Magazine • www.autismparentingmagazine.com
Finding professional resources and guidance can be challenging for families affected by Autism as there is a lot of inconsistent information out there. At *Autism Parenting Magazine*, we aim to provide you with the most current information and interventions so you can make the most informed decisions about what will benefit your child.

Our Autism magazine is suitable for parents of children with Asperger's, PDD-NOS, or Kanner's Autism. We also have a large number of parents who are on the spectrum.

PBS Kids — Sesame Street • autism.sesamestreet.org
Sesame Workshop created Sesame Street and Autism: See Amazing in All Children, a nationwide initiative aimed at communities with children ages two to five. Developed with input from parents, people who serve the Autism community, and people with Autism, See Amazing in All Children offers families ways to manage common challenges, to simplify everyday activities, and to grow connections and support from family, friends, and community.

RESOURCES

Velcro Shoes (blog) • www.velcro-shoes.com
A place to share, a place to feel connected, and a place to be vulnerable and real. No judgment.

"I am in practice to be vulnerable and authentic. I am sharing stories as an outlet, but also to remind us all that we are not alone. I am a talker and a sharer of experience. I learn from listening. I share my kids struggles, the programs we have gone through and specialists we have seen. I am proud of my children...not speaking about their obstacles or diagnosis doesn't change who they are. If I can help just one person by sharing my stories, whether it helps them find direction or just feel connected, I will."

— Alli Baldocchi

We are Brave Together • www.wearebravetogether.com
We Are Brave Together is a nonprofit organization that provides respite, community, and mentoring for mothers caring for children of any age with disabilities, special needs, or other medical or mental health challenges.

Life with a Side of Spectrum — Instagram
Shannon Biancamano, blogger, published photographer.

Regional, Local Organizations and Services

Our Village • www.ourvillageslc.org • Redondo Beach, CA 90278
Mission: to help children, teenagers, and young adults with Autism by providing social skills groups that are research-based and offer exceptional quality for families. Includes **Sibling Support Groups and PEERS Social Skills Groups.**

Shoreline Speech and Language • www.shorelinespeech.com • Hermosa Beach, CA
A small, therapist-owned, pediatric clinic where we understand that no two children are alike. We develop treatment plans for your children that are tailored to meet their own needs and learning style to ensure the best opportunity for success.

Jenny Friedman, Dietitian Nutritionist • www.JennyFriedmanNutrition.com
She teaches Autistic kids to try new foods while giving their parents practical strategies to improve diet variety and nutrition, so they stress less, enjoy family meals, and finally feel confident feeding their child.

The Friendship Foundation • www.friendshipfoundation.com • Redondo Beach, CA
The Friendship Foundation supports parents and families who have children and young adults with special

needs by providing a safe, accepting, and inclusive environment where they can enjoy sports, art, music, and many other social programs with their peers. Our friendly staff and helpful volunteers create a fun experience for all. It is our belief that every person is precious and capable of love, connection, and friendship.

Neuro Fit Systems • www.neuro-fit.com • Los Angeles, CA
A non-medical approach to address the foundational element of neuropathway efficiency.

Neurozone Inc • www.neurozonewave.com •
Playa Del Rey, CA
Optimizing brain function with integrated therapies — Neurofeedback.

Play Sense • www.playsensekids.com •
Los Angeles South Bay
Playing to Learn & Learning to Play. Provides occupational therapy services to children, teens, and young adults.

Play 2 Learn • Cognitive Behavior Therapy (CBT) • www.p2Lfamilytherapy.com
Play Therapy, a modality of child therapy, is a powerful tool for addressing cognitive, behavioral, and emotional challenges. The vehicle of play is used therapeutically to help clients better process their experiences and develop more effective strategies for managing their inner and external worlds.

Educational Therapy Services • www.edtherapy.co • Torrance, CA
Academic, social, and emotional support for students K-12.

Neuropsychologist • www.attentionandlearningservices.com • Torrance, CA
Psychodiagnostics assessment and testing — developmental diagnostic assessment — individual and family psychotherapy — developmental psychotherapy — parent education and support — cogmed working memory training.

The Right Side of Learning • www.therightsideoflearning.com
The Right Side of Learning shows your child how to approach schoolwork. Our strategies strengthen long-term memory, attention skills, ability to learn independently, and test taking skills.

FirstSteps for Kids • www.firststepsforkids.com
FirstSteps for Kids, Inc. specializes in improving the lives of children diagnosed with Autism and related developmental and behavioral disorders. With expertise in applied behavior analysis, our FirstSteps team is prepared to provide your child with effective and comprehensive treatment intervention tailored to address your child's individual needs.

RESOURCES

Surfers Healing • www.Surfershealing.org
Surfers Healing is the original surf camp for children with Autism, and we've been serving the community since 1996. Yet what we offer isn't a "cure" or even "traditional" therapy. It's a completely different sensation and environment for our participants. We give individuals a chance to encounter the waves, to challenge themselves, to try something new.

A.skate Foundation • askate.org
The A.skate Foundation is an organization that allows children with Autism to be a part of our social world through skateboarding. We hold clinics for children with Autism at no cost to the families, give grants to children with Autism for skateboard gear, as well as promote awareness and educate families about the skateboard industry. Autism, like skateboarding, can be unpredictable and often times unruly. We embrace the parts of Autism that are hard to understand and give these kids an outlet that is free of rules or judgment and allows them to be social without being "social."

Ride to Fly • www.ridetofly.com
Therapeutic horseback riding — a nonprofit organization dedicated to providing therapeutic horseback riding and the associated learning experiences to children and adults with disabilities in a safe, nurturing environment. We believe in the inherent worth and dignity of all people and wish to share the special gift of horsemanship with those with special needs.

**Disabled Sports Eastern Sierra •
disabledsportseasternsierra.org**
Nonprofit organization providing adaptive sports and therapeutic outdoor recreation for people with disabilities. Providing programs for people of all ages with physical and/or intellectual disabilities to have fun, healthy, inspiring experiences outdoors in the beautiful Eastern Sierra. Program runs summer and winter.

ABOUT THE AUTHOR

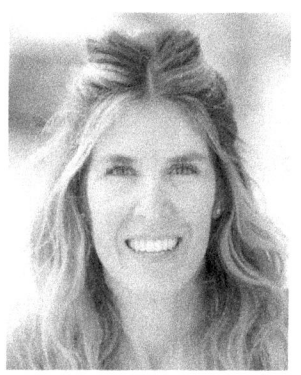

I *am an Autism Mom*. That took me years of tears and confusion, laughter, and pain, fighting and advocating, plus rationalizing and self-blame… to say and really feel. It wasn't because I was ashamed or secretive about my son's diagnosis, I was actually very loud and proud. As parents of special needs kids, we want to protect them from the label. I too was afraid to let this label, this "Autism Mom" define me, become me, swallow me whole. And just as I have treated my son as a person, as a kid, as CADEN, not as an Autistic being, I have learned that I am Alli, I am me. And yes, I am an Autism Mom, but I am so much more.

My careers in fashion, teaching, real estate, and interior styling, were not a waste. I have taken bits and pieces from each career, each step in my journey, to help me grow and arrive where I am today. I am a present, living my life with purpose. I feel and I love. Every small moment is noticed, and I continue to grow with each breath I take. I have joy and gratitude. I have come so far and know I have a long way to go, but I trust that I am exactly where I am supposed to be today.

Now I share this journey and help others on theirs. Sitting in a place of overwhelm, not having a direction can be paralyzing. Your life can be different if you have someone guiding you, giving you the tools, you needed to bring back joy to your everyday life with unshakable confidence, clarity, and purpose. You can become your future self. I did and you can too! *I am an autism mom and so much more!*

www.ingramcontent.com/pod-product-compliance
Lightning Source LLC
Chambersburg PA
CBHW071346080526
44587CB00017B/2979